Strategies, Techniques, & Approaches to Thinking

Case Studies in Clinical Nursing

Second edition

Sandra Luz Martinez de Castillo, EdD, RN
Instructor, Department of Nursing
Contra Costa College
San Pablo, California

SAUNDERS
An Imprint of Elsevier

SAUNDERS
An Imprint of Elsevier

11830 Westline Industrial Drive
St. Louis, MO 63146

Strategies, Techniques, and Approaches to Thinking:
Case Studies in Clinical Nursing

ISBN 0-7216-9772-0

Notice

Pharmacology is an ever-changing field. Standard safety precautions must be followed, but as new research and clinical experience broaden our knowledge, changes in treatment and drug therapy may become necessary or appropriate. Readers are advised to check the most current product information provided by the manufacturer of each drug to be administered to verify the recommended dose, the method and duration of administration, and contraindications. It is the responsibility of the licensed prescriber, relying on experience and knowledge of the patient, to determine dosages and the best treatment for each individual patient. Neither the publisher nor the editor assumes any liability for any injury and/or damage to persons or property arising from this publication.

The Publisher

Vice President, Publishing Director: Sally Schrefer
Executive Editor: Michael S. Ledbetter
Senior Developmental Editor: Laurie K. Muench
Project Manager: Gayle May Morris
Designer: Theresa Breckwoldt

WB/MV

Printed in the United States of America

Last digit is the print number: 9 8 7 6 5 4

PREFACE

Dear Nursing Student:

Nursing is such a wonderful profession. It not only provides you with the opportunity to practice in the acute care setting, but it also allows you to branch off into other career paths, such as teaching, flight nursing, administrative work, or home health nursing – just to name a few. During the next several months, you will be learning many of the nursing concepts, principles, and skills necessary to function in the clinical setting. An important part of your learning is to apply critical thinking skills to help you make sound clinical decisions. This manual is designed to assist you to develop critical thinking skills and to provide you with practice in reading and answering higher level thinking test questions.

The manual is divided into five sections to coincide with your learning needs. Because it is very important to have a strong theoretical foundation, **Section One** is devoted to reinforcing concepts and principles pertinent to nursing practice. Knowledge is fundamental to using critical thinking skills, so take your time and work through the case studies and the learning activities. Every effort was made to develop short clinical case studies and patient care situations that are encountered in the clinical setting. The case studies in Section One have a dual purpose: (1) to reinforce fundamental concepts and principles and (2) to demonstrate how learned knowledge is applied in patient care situations.

Section Two is devoted to helping you prioritize and make sound clinical decisions. Similar to Section One, the case studies designed for this section focus on common clinical situations. You are encouraged to discuss and compare your decisions and rationales with your peers and your instructor. The discussion process is very important. It is through the mutual sharing of knowledge, ideas, and experiences that you will learn how to prioritize and make clinical decisions based on sound rationales. The nursing process is included in this section to assist you in applying the components of assessment, nursing diagnosis, planning, and implementation.

Section Three presents clinical situations using an intershift report format. The presenting situation is given through the intershift report. Relevant and irrelevant information is provided in order to assist you to **analyze** and **interpret** data based on the presenting situation. Flow charts in the form of the patient's Nursing Care Rand/Kardex, Medication Record, Intake and Output Record, Nursing Notes, or History and Physical are provided to assist you in gathering further data. This activity helps you, (1) focus on gathering the data, both from the report and the flow charts, and (2) make relevant connections between the data.

Section Four addresses issues related to the development of management and leadership skills. Like other case studies throughout this book, it is important for you to use critical thinking skills to fully discuss and address the main issues of the case studies, make clinical decisions, and evaluate the solutions to the problems encountered in these situations.

Section Five provides you with additional test questions to assist you in testing your knowledge and to help you apply test-taking strategies.

Finally, the **Critical Thinking Model** provides a simple, yet logical format for looking at the case studies. The Critical Thinking Model can be used in any clinical setting to assist you in the process of developing and using critical thinking skills. I hope that you will enjoy working with these activities, that you gain more practice in answering test questions and, most of all, that you enjoy engaging in the learning process!

DEDICATION

Para mi familia – aquí y en el cielo

REVIEWERS

Denyce Watties-Daniels, MS, RN
Assistant Professor of Nursing
Coppin State College
Baltimore, Maryland

Linda Meade Harris, RN, MSN
Nursing Instructor
Cuesta Community College
San Luis Obispo, California

Margaret A. Sutherland, BSN, MSN
Nursing Instructor
Lancaster General Hospital
Lancaster Institute for Health Education
Lebanon, Pennsylvania

ACKNOWLEDGMENT

To all my students—for giving me
the joy of teaching . . .

CONTENTS

Section One - Cognitive-Building Critical Thinking Activities

Section Two - Priority-Setting and Decision-Making Activities

SECTION ONE

Cognitive-Building Critical Thinking Activities

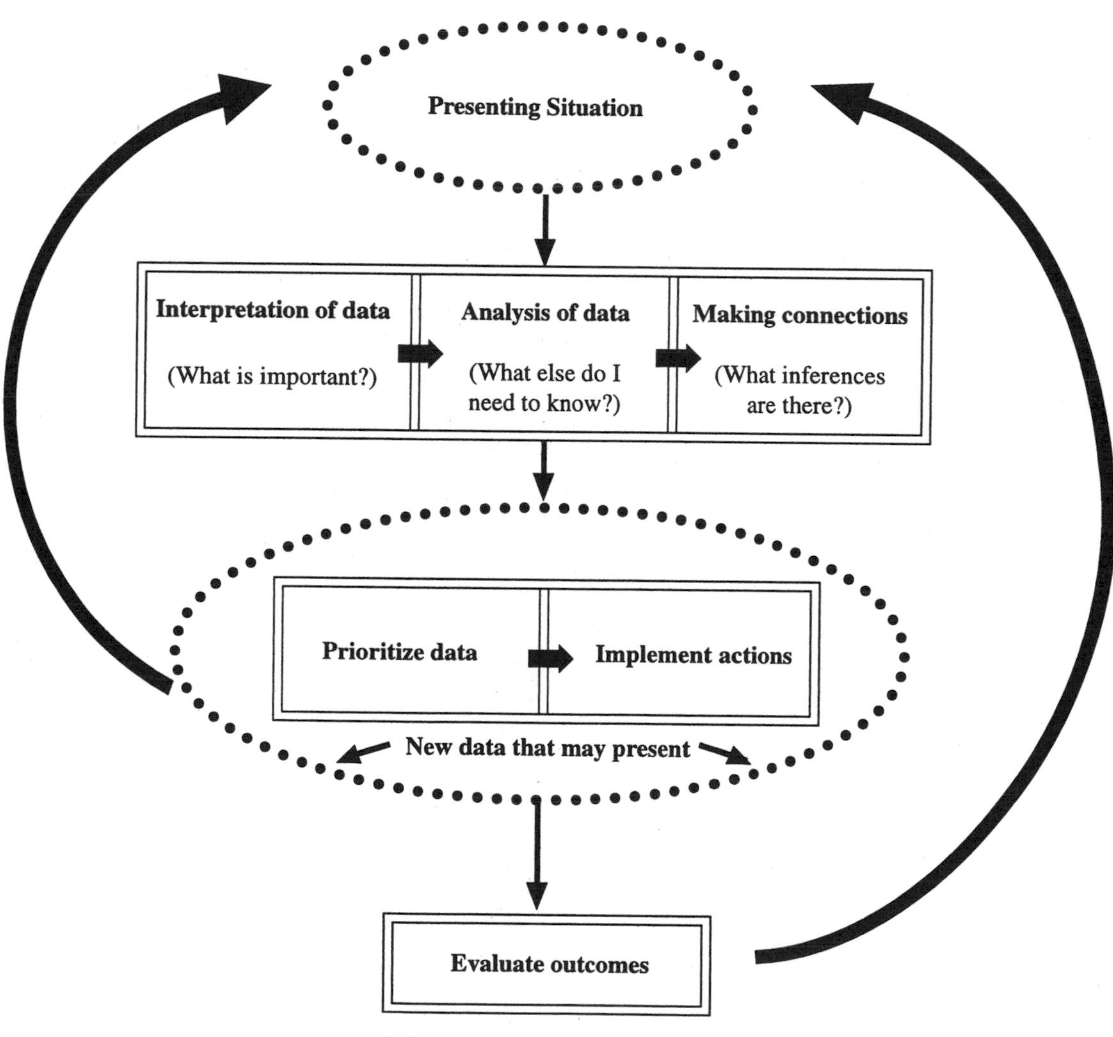

SKIN INTEGRITY

List the **factors** that increase the **risk** of a client developing a pressure ulcer:

1. ______________________
2. ______________________
3. ______________________
4. ______________________
5. ______________________
6. ______________________
7. ______________________
8. ______________________
9. ______________________
10. ______________________
11. ______________________

Use the diagram to **circle** the areas of the body where **pressure ulcers** are likely to develop on a bedridden patient:

Case Study: An 88-year-old female client has been admitted to the hospital with a fractured left elbow. She is malnourished and weighs only 90 lb. She is currently confused and the physician has ordered a vest posey restraint to prevent her from falling out of bed. The client is anorexic and her skin is soft and thin. She is incontinent of urine.

Pertinent Terminology	Definition
Pressure ulcer	
Necrosis	
Ischemia	
Reactive hyperemia	
Blanching	
Slough	
Eschar	
Tunneling	
Debridement	
Excoriation	

Use the case study to **circle the number** that best applies to the client's risk for developing pressure ulcers (the **lower the number**, the greater the risk for the development of pressure ulcers).

Norton's Pressure Area Risk Assessment Form (Scoring System)

General Physical Condition		Mental State		Activity		Mobility		Incontinence		Total Score
Good	4	Alert	4	Ambulatory	4	Full	4	Absent	4	
Fair	3	Apathetic	3	Walks with help	3	Slightly limited	3	Occasional	3	
Poor	2	Confused	2	Chairbound	2	Very limited	2	Usually urinary	2	
Very bad	1	Stuporous	1	Bedbound	1	Immobile	1	Double	1	________

From Norton, D., McLaren, R., Exton-Smith, AN. *An Investigation of Geriatric Nursing Problems in Hospital*. National Corporation for the Care of Old People (now the Centre for Policy on Ageing), London, 1962. Edinburgh: Churchill-Livingstone.

» After 2 days of taking care of the client, the nurse made the following documentation on the client's chart: "Redden, excoriated circular area on sacrum, approximately 2.5 cm × 2.5 cm Dr. Stanley notified."

» Use the documentation to check off (✓) the **"Stage"** of the client's pressure ulcer from the **Pressure Ulcer Stages** below:

Stage 1

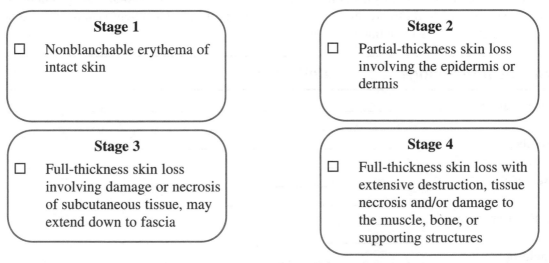

☐ Nonblanchable erythema of intact skin

Stage 2

☐ Partial-thickness skin loss involving the epidermis or dermis

Stage 3

☐ Full-thickness skin loss involving damage or necrosis of subcutaneous tissue, may extend down to fascia

Stage 4

☐ Full-thickness skin loss with extensive destruction, tissue necrosis and/or damage to the muscle, bone, or supporting structures

Interactive Activity: With a partner, **write in** the **"Stage"** of the pressure ulcer for each of the following case studies using the **Pressure Ulcer Stages**:

Case Study	Pressure Ulcer Stage
A male client was brought into the hospital. He has an open wound on his left heel that is 2″ wide and ½″ deep. It has a foul odor and the heel bone is exposed.	________________
The nurse measures an irregular open wound on the right hip. The subcutaneous tissue is visible.	________________

Applying Critical Thinking Skills to Test Questions

INSTRUCTIONS: Circle the one best answer for each test question. Write your rationale for selecting the answer. To enhance your learning and test taking skill, discuss your answer and rationale with a partner. The answer and the rationale can be found on the back of this page.

1. The nurse is taking care of a client who has a Stage 1 pressure ulcer on the sacrum. In delegating the care of the client, it is most important for the nurse to
   a. instruct the nursing assistant to turn the client q2h.
   b. ask the nursing assistant to massage the client's sacrum.
   c. review how to assess the client's sacrum with the nursing assistant.
   d. inform the nursing assistant of the client's pressure ulcer.

   Rationale for your selection: ____

2. While reading the chart of a client, the nurse notes that the physician has identified eschar on the left heel. Which of the following assessments is most significant of this finding?
   a. A black scabbed-like area on the left heel
   b. A bruised area on the left heel
   c. A Stage 3 pressure ulcer on the left heel
   d. A Stage 4 pressure ulcer on the left heel

   Rationale for your selection: ____

3. Upon turning a client to the lateral position the nurse notes a reddened area on the right hip. Further assessment reveals intact skin with blanching at the site. Which of the following is the most appropriate nursing intervention?
   a. Notify the physician.
   b. Document the findings.
   c. Apply a dry sterile dressing.
   d. Document the presence of a Stage 1 pressure ulcer.

   Rationale for your selection: ____

Applying Critical Thinking Skills to Test Questions

HELPFUL HINTS: Read all test questions carefully. Identify key words in the question that will guide you in answering the question. In these test questions the **key words** to consider are "**most important**," "**most significant**," and "**most appropriate**." Compare your rationale with the one in the test question.

1. The nurse is taking care of a client who has a Stage 1 pressure ulcer on the sacrum. In delegating the care of the client, it is most important for the nurse to
   (a.) instruct the nursing assistant to turn the client q2h.
   b. ask the nursing assistant to massage the client's sacrum.
   c. review how to assess the client's sacrum with the nursing assistant.
   d. inform the nursing assistant of the client's pressure ulcer.

   Rationale: **(A) is the answer. Instructing the nursing assistant to carry out an intervention that would assist in preventing further skin breakdown is most important. Option (b) could cause more tissue damage; option (c) is not appropriate for a nursing assistant to assess, and option (d) is not client centered nor provides a specific intervention to assist the client.**

2. While reading the chart of a client, the nurse notes that the physician has identified eschar on the left heel. Which of the following assessments is most significant of this finding?
   (a.) A black scabbed-like area on the left heel
   b. A bruised area on the left heel
   c. A Stage 3 pressure ulcer on the left heel
   d. A Stage 4 pressure ulcer on the left heel

   Rationale: **(A) is the answer. Describes the appearance of eschar. Eschar must be debrided to "stage" the pressure ulcer. Options (b), (c), and (d) do not describe the finding.**

3. Upon turning a client to the lateral position the nurse notes a reddened area on the right hip. Further assessment reveals intact skin with blanching at the site. Which of the following is the most appropriate nursing intervention?
   a. Notify the physician.
   (b) Document the findings.
   c. Apply a dry sterile dressing.
   d. Document the presence of a Stage 1 pressure ulcer.

   Rationale: **(B) is the answer. A reddened area with intact skin and blanching indicates circulation to the site. Options (a) and (c) are not necessary at this time. For option (d), the findings do not support the definition of a Stage 1 pressure ulcer.**

Applying Critical Thinking Skills to Test Questions

INSTRUCTIONS: Circle the one best answer for each test question. Write your rationale for selecting the answer. To enhance your learning and test-taking skill, discuss your answer and rationale with a partner. The answer and the rationale can be found on the back of this page.

1. The following conversation takes place at the client's bedside:
   Nurse: "Good morning Mr. J., I am your nurse for today. Did you sleep well?"
   Client: "I am not sure."
   Nurse: "You are not sure?"
   Which of the following statements is most accurate of this conversation? The nurse
   a. should ask a question to validate the client's confusion.
   b. used an appropriate follow-up communication technique.
   c. should look at the chart to see how the client slept.
   d. was inappropriate in asking the second question.

   Rationale for your selection: ____________________
   ____
   ____
   ____
   ____

2. The nurse walks into a client's room and sees the postsurgical client holding his abdomen and grimacing. The nurse states "You look like you are in pain."
   The nurse's statement is
   a. appropriate because it states what the nurse is observing.
   b. appropriate because pain is expected after surgery.
   c. inappropriate because the nurse made a conclusion before validating.
   d. inappropriate because the nurse should wait for the client to speak first.

   Rationale for your selection: ____________________
   ____
   ____
   ____
   ____

3. The following conversation takes place at the client's bedside:
   Nurse: "Mr. T, I will be teaching you how to change your surgical dressing."
   Client: "I would prefer that you wait until my wife gets here. She takes care of everything."
   Nurse: "You shouldn't depend on your wife. I'll show you first, then you can teach your wife."
   The nurse's last statement is
   a. displaying a value judgment.
   b. appropriate because it encourages self-care.
   c. having the client reinforce what will be taught.
   d. inappropriate because that nurse should have called the wife first.

   Rationale for your selection: ____________________
   ____
   ____
   ____
   ____

Applying Critical Thinking Skills to Test Questions

HELPFUL HINTS: Read all test questions carefully. Identify key words in the question that will guide you in answering the question. In these test questions the **key words** to consider are **"most accurate,"** and **"most important."** Compare your rationale with the one in the test question.

1. The following conversation takes place at the client's bedside:
   Nurse: "Good morning Mr. J., I am your nurse for today. Did you sleep well?"
   Client: "I am not sure."
   Nurse: "You are not sure?"

   Which of the following statements is most accurate of this conversation? The nurse
   a. should ask a question to validate the client's confusion.
   (b) used an appropriate follow-up communication technique.
   c. should look at the chart to see how the client slept.
   d. was inappropriate in asking the second question.

   Rationale: **(B) is the answer. The nurse used a reflective (paraphrase) technique to solicit more information from the client. Options (a), (c), and (d) do not solicit more information.**

2. The nurse walks into a client's room and sees the postsurgical client holding his abdomen and grimacing. The nurse states "You look like you are in pain."
   The nurse's statement is
   (a) appropriate because it states what the nurse is observing.
   b. appropriate because pain is expected after surgery.
   c. inappropriate because the nurse made a conclusion before validating.
   d. inappropriate because the nurse should wait for the client to speak first.

   Rationale: **(A) is the answer. The nurse is stating the objective observations. This allows the client to clarify or validate the observation. Options (b), (c), and (d) are not appropriate therapeutic communication techniques that facilitate client communication.**

3. The following conversation takes place at the client's bedside:
   Nurse: "Mr. T, I will be teaching you how to change your surgical dressing."
   Client: "I would prefer that you wait until my wife gets here. She takes care of everything."
   Nurse: "You shouldn't depend on your wife. I'll show you first, then you can teach your wife."
   The nurse's last statement is
   (a) displaying a value judgment.
   b. appropriate because it encourages self-care.
   c. having the client reinforce what will be taught.
   d. inappropriate because that nurse should have called the wife first.

   Rationale: **(A) is the answer. The nurse's comment reflects how the nurse feels about the client's decision. This can cause a block to communication. Options (b), (c), and (d) do not take into consideration the importance of the client's personal needs and social structure.**

REPORTING PATIENT STATUS

List the most common methods nurses use to **report patient status** during the shift and from shift to shift:

1. ______________________
2. ______________________
3. ______________________
4. ______________________

Place an "X" in the box(es) that best describes the information that should be included in a **change of shift report**. The change of shift report should:

- ☐ Provide basic information such as room number, date of admission, and medical diagnosis.
- ☐ Provide specific information regarding the client's needs.
- ☐ Provide information on significant changes in the client's condition.
- ☐ Provide information on follow-up client care.
- ☐ Provide information on clients transferred or discharged from the unit (varies in some hospitals).

Case Study: 0700 (morning audiotaped report on the following two patients)

"Mr. J in room 461 is a 76-year-old man. He was admitted last night with sepsis. He has an IV of D5W infusing at 75 cc/hr. He is NPO. His output for the shift is 150 cc total. The 0600 temperature is 100.6° F and his blood pressure is 146/94.

Mr. H in room 462 has been here for 3 days with pneumonia. His temperature at 0600 was 102.4° F and I gave him 2 Tylenol tablets. He has an IV infusing at 100 cc/hr and there are 300 cc left. He has a productive cough and is bringing up thick whitish phlegm. I sent the sputum specimen to the laboratory. He has taken in only 50 cc of oral fluid and his output was 275 cc for the shift."

Pertinent Terminology	Definition
Nursing Rand/Kardex	
Worksheet	
Reporting	

Use the **case study** to fill in the worksheet with the pertinent information obtained in morning report on the clients:

Worksheet

Pt. Name: ____________ Age: ____________ VS: ____________ ____________ Amb. ______ Bed rest _____ Bath (self) ____ (Bed) _____	Rm: ______ I = ______ O = ______ Diet: ______	Dx: ____________ Admit date ________ IV: ____________ ____________ ____________	Follow-up Notes: ____________ ____________ ____________ ____________ ____________ ____________
Pt. Name: ____________ Age: ____________ VS: ____________ ____________ Amb. ______ Bed rest _____ Bath (self) ____ (Bed) _____	Rm: ______ I = ______ O = ______ Diet: ______	Dx: ____________ Admit date ________ IV: ____________ ____________ ____________	Follow-up Notes: ____________ ____________ ____________ ____________ ____________ ____________

Additional information to **complete the worksheet is found** in the ____________________.

Interactive Activity: With a partner, answer the questions regarding (1) the **change of shift report** for the following case study and (2) **fill in the worksheet** and discuss the **Follow-up Notes**:

1500 (**change of shift** audiotaped report)
"Mr. W, 92 years old, in room 357 was admitted yesterday with anemia. His hemoglobin (Hgb) this morning is 7.2 mg/dl and his hematocrit (Hct) is 26%. He is hard of hearing and weighs 127 lb. His Foley drained only 100 cc all shift. He has an IV of normal saline infusing at 75 cc/hr. He will receive two units of blood this evening. The lab will call when the blood is ready. The family and client will make a decision soon regarding his code status. He is very weak and needs a lot of assistance."

- **Identify the basic information** given in the report: ____________________
____

- **Identify the significant information** given in the report: ____________________
____
____

Worksheet

Pt. Name: ____________ Age: ____________ VS: ____________ ____________ Amb. ______ Bed rest _____ Bath (self) ____ (Bed) _____	Rm: ______ I = ______ O = ______ Diet: ______	Dx: ____________ Admit date ________ IV: ____________ ____________ ____________	Follow-up Notes: ____________ ____________ ____________ ____________ ____________ ____________

INTRODUCTION TO THE ASSESSMENT PROCESS

List the **methods** available to the nurse for the **collection of patient data**:

1. ____________________
2. ____________________
3. ____________________
4. ____________________

List the **parts of the patient's chart** that assist the nurse in the **collection of patient data**:

1. ____________________
2. ____________________
3. ____________________
4. ____________________
5. ____________________
6. ____________________

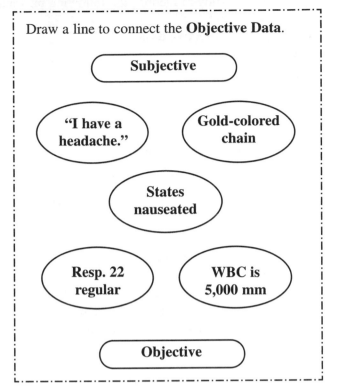

Draw a line to connect the **Objective Data**.

Subjective

"I have a headache."

Gold-colored chain

States nauseated

Resp. 22 regular

WBC is 5,000 mm

Objective

Case Study: Mrs. C has been admitted to the hospital for the birth of her baby. Her husband is by her side. You observe that she is very pleasant but cries out with each contraction. She tells you "I feel a lot of pressure in my back." Her chart indicates that she is 26 years old and that she has a 6-year-old son.

Pertinent Terminology	Definition
Assessment	____________________
Subjective data	____________________
Objective data	____________________
Clustering data	____________________
Validation of data	____________________
Primary source	____________________
Secondary source	____________________

Use the case study to identify the following information:

✎ List the **objective data**: — **Source (Primary/Secondary)**

1. ______________________________
2. ______________________________ ______________
3. ______________________________ ______________
4. ______________________________ ______________

✎ List the **subjective data**:

1. ______________________________ ______________

Interactive Activity: With a partner, **use the box to identify subjective and objective data** from the case studies:

Mrs. T has been admitted with depression. She answers questions softly with a "yes" or "no" response. She wants her door closed and her room dark. She refuses visitors and eats only 10% of her meals. You noticed that she cries regularly and sleeps a lot. She bites her nails frequently.

Objective Data

- ______________________
- ______________________
- ______________________
- ______________________
- ______________________
- ______________________
- ______________________

Subjective Data

- ______________________
- ______________________

Mr. P had surgery 1 day ago. He tells you that he has been very independent all his life and hates being sick. He has refused his pain medication all morning. You notice that he refuses to get out of bed, he moans quietly every now and then, he is sweaty, and his hands are clenched tightly. His surgical dressing is clean and he says everything is fine when you ask him a question.

Objective Data

- ______________________
- ______________________
- ______________________
- ______________________
- ______________________
- ______________________
- ______________________

Subjective Data

- ______________________
- ______________________

Mr. K informs the nursing assistant that he is nauseated. He has refused his lunch. You go in to check him and you notice 100 cc of clear yellow emesis. He tells you that he vomited. His wife is at his bedside.

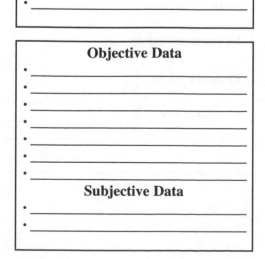

Objective Data

- ______________________
- ______________________
- ______________________
- ______________________
- ______________________
- ______________________
- ______________________

Subjective Data

- ______________________
- ______________________

BASIC PHYSICAL ASSESSMENT

List the **four methods of examination** used in the performance of a physical assessment:

1. ______________________
2. ______________________
3. ______________________
4. ______________________

Write in the most appropriate **method of examination(s)** for each of the following:

- Oral mucous membranes ______________________
- Peripheral pulses ______________________
- Arterial blood pressure ______________________
- Lung sounds ______________________
- Lower extremity edema ______________________
- Apical pulse ______________________
- Distended abdomen ______________________

Case Study: Carrie is a nursing student and is assigned to Ms. W. Ms. W, 18 years old, came to the ER with complaints of right lower abdominal pains. She was admitted and had an appendectomy the day of admission. She is 2 days post-op and will be going home this afternoon. Carrie performs a **body systems assessment** and documents the following notes:

Neuro: Alert and oriented ×3. **Cardiovascular (CV):** Radial pulse regular and bounding. **Skin:** warm and dry, pallor present, turgor elastic. **Respirations (Resp.):** Regular, clear. **Gastrointestinal (GI):** Bowel sounds present in all four quadrants. RLQ abdominal dressing clean, complains of tenderness with palpation. **Genitourinary (GU):** States voiding without difficulty. **Musculoskeletal (MS):** Ambulates with a steady gait. **Psychosocial:** Cheerful.

Pertinent Terminology	Definition
Inspection	
Palpation	
Percussion	
Auscultation	
Chief complaint (CC)	
Review of systems	

Use the documentation notes from the case study to **identify the method of examination** used by Carrie in performing the body systems assessment:

Documentation	Method(s) of Examination
• **Neuro:** Alert and oriented ×3	______________
• **CV:** Radial pulse regular and bounding	______________
• **Skin:** Warm and dry, pallor, turgor elastic	______________
• **Resp.:** Regular, clear	______________
• **GI:** Bowel sounds present in all four quadrants. Right lower quadrant abdominal dressing clean complains of tenderness with palpation	______________
• **GU:** States voiding without difficulty	______________
• **MS:** Ambulates with a steady gait	______________
• **Psychosocial:** Cheerful	______________

Interactive Activity: With a partner, use the following documentation notes to **(1) identify** the **body system** being assessed and **(2) the method of examination** used:

Documentation Notes	Body System/Method(s) of Examination
States it is 1945, does not know where he is; knows first name; hand grips unequal right < left	______________ ______________
Voided 50 cc of amber fluid; abdomen distended	______________ ______________
Warm, moist; pallor with erythema on sacral area; edema 1+ on bilateral lower extremities	______________ ______________
Absent bowel sounds in lower and upper right quadrants, hyperactive on upper and lower left quadrant; having small amounts of liquid dark brown stools	______________ ______________
Wheezes audible on inspiration, coughing, expectorating thick yellowish phlegm.	______________ ______________
Apical pulse 116, rapid, irregular Radial pulse 98, rapid, thready, irregular	______________ ______________
Passive ROM to right hand. Unable to extend and flex fingers	______________ ______________
Left facial drooping; left arm and leg flaccid	______________ ______________

Applying Critical Thinking Skills to Test Questions

INSTRUCTIONS: Circle the one best answer for each test question. Write your rationale for selecting the answer. To enhance your learning and test-taking skill, discuss your answer and rationale with a partner. The answer and the rationale can be found on the back of this page.

1. The nurse is preparing to assess the neuro status of an adult client who had a hip fracture 5 days ago and was reported to have experienced confusion the previous shift. Which statement will provide the nurse with the most appropriate information?
   a. "Can you tell me today's date."
   b. "Do you know that you are in the hospital?"
   c. "When did you have hip surgery?"
   d. "What is your name?"

   Rationale for your selection: ____

   ____

   ____

   ____

   ____

   ____

2. The nurse is informed that a newly admitted client is complaining of itching and has a rash all over the body. The most appropriate nursing intervention initially is to
   a. inform the doctor of the objective and subjective complaints.
   b. inspect the client and describe the rash.
   c. ask the client to try not to scratch the areas.
   d. check the medication record for anti-itch medication.

   Rationale for your selection: ____

   ____

   ____

   ____

   ____

   ____

3. The nurse is assigned to a client who was admitted for a blood clot in the right leg. Which of the following describes the appropriate assessment technique initially?
   a. inspection of the right leg
   b. light palpation of the right leg
   c. inspection followed by deep palpation of edematous areas
   d. light palpation followed by inspection of any reddened areas

   Rationale for your selection: ____

   ____

   ____

   ____

   ____

   ____

Applying Critical Thinking Skills to Test Questions

HELPFUL HINTS: Read all test questions carefully. Identify key words in the question that will guide you in answering the question. In these test questions the **key words** to consider are **"most appropriate"** and **"initially."** Compare your rationale with the one in the test question.

1. The nurse is preparing to assess the neuro status of an adult client who had a hip fracture 5 days ago and was reported to have experienced confusion the previous shift. Which statement will provide the nurse with the most appropriate information?
   a. "Can you tell me today's date."
   b. "Do you know that you are in the hospital?"
   c. "When did you have hip surgery?"
   (d) "What is your name?"

   Rationale: **(D) is the answer. Eliciting orientation to person is part of assessing client orientation. Options (a) and (b) encourage a "yes" or "no" response, and option (c) may not give accurate data if the client does not remember the date.**

2. The nurse is informed that a newly admitted client is complaining of itching and has a rash all over the body. The most appropriate nursing intervention initially is to
   a. inform the doctor of the objective and subjective complaints.
   (b) inspect the client and describe the rash.
   c. ask the client to try not to scratch the areas.
   d. check the medication record for anti-itch medication.

   Rationale: **(B) is the answer. It is most appropriate for the nurse to initially gather data by using the assessment skill of inspection and then to further describe the observations. Options (a), (c), and (d) are follow-up nursing interventions.**

3. The nurse is assigned to a client who was admitted for a blood clot in the right leg. Which of the following describes the appropriate assessment technique initially?
   (a.) inspection of the right leg
   b. light palpation of the right leg
   c. inspection followed by deep palpation of edematous areas
   d. light palpation followed by inspection of any reddened areas

   Rationale: **(A) is the answer. Inspection is the initial step in the assessment process that provides information on color, size, shape, and movement of the extremity. Options (b) and (d) are not appropriate initially and option (c) should not be done in this situation.**

SELF-CONCEPT

List the **four components** of **self-concept**:

1. ______________________
2. ______________________
3. ______________________
4. ______________________

For each of the **self-concept** components **identify two stressors** that affect and contribute to altering the component of:

- **Identity** (any two)

  ____

  ____

- **Body image** (any two)

  ____

  ____

  ____

- **Self-esteem** (any two)

  ____

  ____

  ____

- **Role performance** (any two)

  ____

  ____

Case Study: A female client was diagnosed with breast cancer 2 weeks ago and recently had a left mastectomy. She is 32 years old and is married with a 5-year-old daughter. She is very anxious after the surgery and wonders how her husband will react to her. She tells the nurse: "I am so young to have this done." She begins to cry and says that she loves being a mom, but doesn't think she can have another child because she would not be able to nurse and care for the baby as she would like to. She is scheduled to begin chemotherapy treatments in 1 week.

Pertinent Terminology	Definition
Self-concept	
Identity	
Body image	
Self-esteem	
Role performance	

Reread the case study and cluster the **objective data** and **subjective data** that relate to the **self-concept** component that is marked with an "**X**":

- ☐ Identity
- ☒ **Body image**
- ☐ Self-esteem
- ☐ Role performance

➨ **Objective data:**

____

____

____

➨ **Subjective data:**

____

____

- ☐ Identity
- ☐ Body image
- ☐ Self-esteem
- ☒ **Role performance**

➨ **Objective data:**

____

____

____

____

____

➨ **Subjective data:**

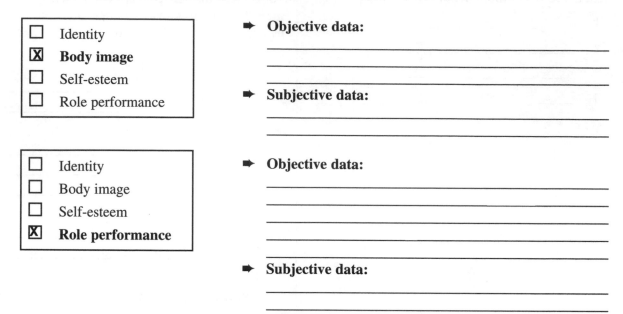

____

____

Interactive Activity: With a partner, use the following case study to cluster the objective data and the subjective data related to the **self-concept** component that is marked with an "**X**":

CASE STUDY

A male client suffered a heart attack 2 months ago and has lost his job. When he comes to the clinic, his facial expression is tense and he speaks in a hostile voice. During the last visit, he stated: "I can't just sit here, I am the breadwinner of my family." "I'm useless since I had the heart attack!"

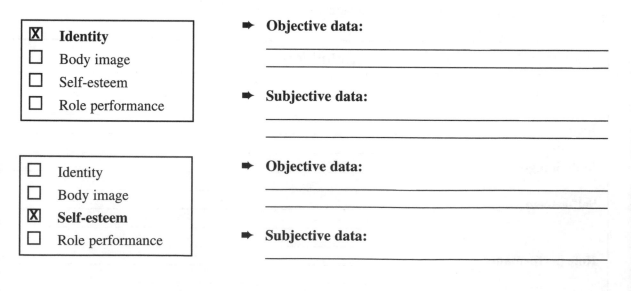

- ☒ **Identity**
- ☐ Body image
- ☐ Self-esteem
- ☐ Role performance

➨ **Objective data:**

____

____

➨ **Subjective data:**

____

____

- ☐ Identity
- ☐ Body image
- ☒ **Self-esteem**
- ☐ Role performance

➨ **Objective data:**

____

____

➨ **Subjective data:**

____

CULTURAL ASPECTS OF NURSING

List the **six cultural phenomena** that influence nursing care:

1. ______________________
2. ______________________
3. ______________________
4. ______________________
5. ______________________
6. ______________________

List **two examples** for each of the following:

Communication

1. ______________________
2. ______________________

Social organizations

1. ______________________
2. ______________________

Environmental control

1. ______________________
2. ______________________

Biological variations

1. ______________________
2. ______________________

Case Study: Wendy RN, the home health nurse, visits a 62-year-old Hispanic woman who has had diabetes mellitus for 20 years and currently has a sore on her left foot. The client has missed two of her doctor's appointments and has been soaking her foot in warm salt water every night. The client speaks English but does not like to call the clinic or question the nurse because she does want to bother anyone. She enjoys cooking and eating Mexican food. During the home visit Wendy noticed several religious artifacts and many pictures of the client's children and grandchildren on the wall.

Pertinent Terminology	Definition
Culture	
Culture shock	
Cultural sensitivity	
Ethnicity	
Acculturation	
Ethnocentrism	
Transcultural nursing	

Use the case study to **identify** the **cultural data** that relates to the **culture phenomena** listed below:

Culture Phenomena	Cultural Data
Communication	______________________
Space	______________________
Time	______________________
Social organization	______________________
Environmental control	______________________
Biological variation	______________________

Interactive Activity: With a partner, use the following case studies to (1) **underline** the pertinent **cultural data** and (2) **identify** the **possible implications** for health care delivery:

Case Study	Health Care Delivery Implication(s)
A Filipino woman, is very quiet. She rarely complains and the nurses comment on how she doesn't maintain eye contact when the nurse is speaking.	______________________
A client of Chinese ancestry is 80 years old and requires constant care. She lives with one of her daughters and all of the adult family members are involved in caring for her at night.	______________________
Mrs. W has had a miscarriage. She hemorrhaged and her blood count is very low. The physician has recommended a blood transfusion, but Mrs. W refuses because of her religious beliefs.	______________________
An African-American woman comes to the outpatient clinic for blood pressure checks. She tells the nurse that her youngest daughter is about to be married. She is concerned because her other daughter has sickle cell anemia.	______________________
A male client had major surgery yesterday. He does not want to get out of bed and has refused all his pain medication. The nurse knows that he is in pain but wants to respect his wishes.	______________________

Applying Critical Thinking Skills to Test Questions

INSTRUCTIONS: Circle the one best answer for each test question. Write your rationale for selecting the answer. To enhance your learning and test-taking skill, discuss your answer and rationale with a partner. The answer and the rationale can be found on the back of this page.

1. The nurse is asking an alert elderly Hispanic female client to sign a consent for a bronchoscopy procedure scheduled the next day. The client tells that nurse that she wants to wait until her family arrives later. Which nursing action is most appropriate?
   a. Ask the client to sign; but inform her that she can change her mind.
   b. Ask the client if she has any questions you can answer.
   c. Tell the client to call you when her family arrives.
   d. Inform the doctor.

   Rationale for your selection: ______________________________
   ____
   ____
   ____
   ____
   ____

2. The nurse is taking care of a client who is scheduled for surgery today. The client asks the nurse to read a passage from the Bible to help her prepare herself for surgery. It is most appropriate for the nurse to
   a. read the Bible passage.
   b. ask if someone on staff is the same religion as the client.
   c. kindly tell the client that nurses cannot get involved in religious issues.
   d. inquire if the client would prefer that a religious person be called.

   Rationale for your selection: ______________________________
   ____
   ____
   ____
   ____
   ____

3. The nurse is assigned to a client who believes that wearing a copper bracelet will relieve arthritic pain. In providing care for the client, it is most important for the nurse to
   a. encourage the client to use anti-inflammatory medication.
   b. inform the client that copper bracelets have no proven medical value.
   c. address the pathophysiology associated with arthritis with the client.
   d. respect the beliefs associated with the copper bracelet by the client..

   Rationale for your selection: ______________________________
   ____
   ____
   ____
   ____
   ____

Applying Critical Thinking Skills to Test Questions

HELPFUL HINTS: Read all test questions carefully. Identify key words in the question that will guide you in answering the question. In these test questions the **key words** to consider are **"most appropriate"** and **"most important."** Compare your rationale with the one in the test question.

1. The nurse is asking an alert elderly Hispanic female client to sign a consent for a bronchoscopy procedure scheduled the next day. The client tells that nurse that she wants to wait until her family arrives later. Which nursing action is most appropriate?
   a. Ask the client to sign; but inform her that she can change her mind.
   b. Ask the client if she has any questions you can answer.
   (c.) Tell the client to call you when her family arrives.
   d. Inform the doctor.

   Rationale: **(C) is the answer. The family is an important social organization in many cultures. Being available when the family arrives is manifesting respect for the client's wishes and cultural sensitivity. Options (a), (b), and (d) do not address cultural sensitivity.**

2. The nurse is taking care of a client who is scheduled for surgery today. The client asks the nurse to read a passage from the Bible to help her prepare herself for surgery. It is most appropriate for the nurse to
   (a.) read the Bible passage.
   b. ask if someone on staff is the same religion as the client.
   c. kindly tell the client that nurses cannot get involved in religious issues.
   d. inquire if the client would prefer that a religious person be called.

   Rationale: **(A) is the answer. Recognizing the spiritual needs of a client is viewing the client as a whole person with spiritual as well as physical needs. Options (b), (c), and (d) defer the needs of the patient to someone else.**

3. The nurse is assigned to a client who believes that wearing a copper bracelet will relieve arthritic pain. In providing care for the client, it is most important for the nurse to
   a. encourage the client to use anti-inflammatory medication.
   b. inform the client that copper bracelets have no proven medical value.
   c. address the pathophysiology associated with arthritis with the client.
   (d.) respect the beliefs associated with the copper bracelet by the client..

   Rationale: **(D) is the answer. Cultural beliefs play an important role in the healing process. This cultural belief does not interfere with the client's well-being. Options (a), (b), and (c) tend to minimize the client's belief.**

INTRODUCTION TO FORMULATING A NURSING DIAGNOSIS

List the **5 steps of the Nursing Process:**

1. ______________________
2. ______________________
3. ______________________
4. ______________________
5. ______________________

The **NANDA Nursing Diagnoses** are classified and formulated to address the client's health problems which can be:

1. ______________________
2. ______________________
3. ______________________
4. ______________________

Circle the **words** that may be used to give specific meaning to the Nursing Diagnosis statement:

Related to
Increased
Altered
Well
Risk for
Acute
Impaired
Sign/Symptom
Due to
Possible

Case Study: The home health nurse makes the following observations and documents the following after visiting a 68-year-old male client: Lives alone, his only son lives 60 miles away, visits monthly and calls weekly. The client stays indoors all day. His vision is poor and he is not able to drive.

Pertinent Terminology	Definition
NANDA	
Nursing process	
Assessment	
Nursing diagnosis	
Defining characteristics	
Planning	
Implementation	
Evaluation	
Etiology	

From the case study, **check off (✓) the Nursing Diagnosis** most appropriate for the client (✸ Use a Nursing Diagnosis book to validate your selection):

Nursing Diagnoses:

__ Coping, ineffective
__ Loneliness, risk for
__ Social isolation

List the **defining characteristics** for the **nursing diagnosis** you selected:

✸ ____________ ✸ ____________ ✸ ____________

✸ ____________ ✸ ____________

☛ **Further documentation** by the home health nurse states: The client has lost 10 lb since the last visit 2 weeks ago. He now is malnourished and lives on a limited income. He needs the services of a nutritionist and a community service that delivers meals to homebound individuals.

From the **further documentation** data, **check off (✓) the Nursing Diagnosis** most appropriate for the client:

Nursing Diagnoses:

__ Social isolation
__ Knowledge, deficient
__ Nutrition, imbalanced: less than body requirements

List the **current pertinent defining characteristics** for the nursing diagnosis you selected:

✸ ____________ ✸ ____________ ✸ ____________

Interactive Activity: With a partner, review the following case studies and **identify** the **defining characteristics** that relate to the **Nursing Diagnosis** written next to each situation.

Case Study	✸ Defining Characteristics
The client has a Stage II pressure ulcer on her right heel. She has been on bed rest and her right leg is elevated.	**SKIN INTEGRITY, IMPAIRED** ✸ ____________
The client has oral lesions in his mouth caused by a treatment of chemotherapy. He complains of pain and his mouth is red.	**ORAL MEMBRANES, IMPAIRED** ✸ ____________ ____________
The client is scheduled for surgery in the morning. She says that she is very scared because her grandmother died during surgery.	**FEAR** ✸ ____________

FORMULATING A NURSING DIAGNOSIS

List the components of the:

Two-part Nursing Diagnosis statement:

1. ______________________
2. ______________________

Three-part Nursing Diagnosis statement:

1. ______________________
2. ______________________
3. ______________________

Place an "X" in the box that identifies the common errors made in the development of the Nursing Diagnosis statement:

- ☐ Using the NANDA diagnostic categories to identify the nursing diagnosis
- ☐ Using the medical diagnosis in the formulation of the nursing diagnosis
- ☐ Clustering the subjective/objective data
- ☐ Using signs and symptoms to write the nursing diagnosis statement
- ☐ Making legally inadvisable statements
- ☐ Misinterpreting the meaning of the subjective and objective data
- ☐ Being very specific in defining the etiology
- ☐ Using qualifying words in the diagnostic statement

Case Study: The client is to be scheduled for elective surgery. In preparation for the surgery, the office nurse takes the client's health history. The nurse documents that the client has recently been diagnosed with diabetes mellitus and was prescribed an antidiabetic pill to take every morning. The client tells the nurse that she stopped the "pill" one week ago because she was feeling better.

Pertinent Terminology	Definition
Nursing diagnosis	
Defining characteristics	
Risk factors	
Etiology	
Data cluster	

Use the **case study** to **cluster the subjective and objective data**:

Objective data: ____

____

Subjective data: ____

☞ Use the data to complete the nursing diagnosis below with a **three-part statement** for the client:

Deficient knowledge: ____

____

Interactive Activity: With a partner, review the following case studies and (1) **list** the **defining characteristics**, (2) **identify the error** in the **nursing diagnosis** statement, and (3) **write a correct nursing diagnosis**:

Case Study

The client has been confused all morning. He has attempted to get OOB and does not know who he is. His laboratory diagnostic studies indicate that he has a decreased serum sodium level. The nurse wrote the following nursing diagnosis:

Defining Characteristics

1. ______________________________
2. ______________________________

Chronic confusion, r/t electrolyte imbalance

Error(s)

1. ______________________________
2. ______________________________

____

3. ______________________________

____

Nursing Diagnosis

____

____

____

____

The client goes weekly to the outpatient clinic to have his blood pressure checked. He smokes one pack of cigarettes per day. His blood pressure is 146/88. His father died from heart disease at age 49, and his brother is recovering from a heart attack. The nurse writes the following nursing diagnosis:

Defining Characteristics

1. ______________________________

____

Risk for heart attack r/t smoking and family history of heart disease

Error(s)

1. ______________________________

____

Nursing Diagnosis

____

____

Applying Critical Thinking Skills to Test Questions

INSTRUCTIONS: Circle the one best answer for each test question. Write your rationale for selecting the answer. To enhance your learning and test-taking skill, discuss your answer and rationale with a partner. The answer and the rationale can be found on the back of this page.

1. The nurse clusters the client's objective and subjective signs and symptoms primarily to
   a. identify the nursing diagnosis.
   b. correlate with the medical diagnosis.
   c. validate the subjective complaints.
   d. work with at "risk for" diagnoses.

   Rationale for your selection: ______________________________
   ____
   ____
   ____
   ____
   ____

2. The following nursing diagnosis is found on the client rand: Hip fracture r/t fall. In evaluating the written diagnosis, the nurse correctly concludes that the diagnosis
   a. is written appropriately.
   b. needs a modifier after the r/t statement.
   c. needs a modifier in the first part of the statement.
   d. is written inappropriately.

   Rationale for your selection: ______________________________
   ____
   ____
   ____
   ____
   ____

3. The nurse admits an elderly client with the medical diagnosis of dehydration. In developing the nursing diagnoses, it is most important for the nurse to
   a. establish nursing diagnoses that are based on the medical diagnosis.
   b. focus on nursing diagnoses that affect fluid balance.
   c. gather data to support actual nursing diagnoses.
   d. include actual and risk for diagnoses.

   Rationale for your selection: ______________________________
   ____
   ____
   ____
   ____
   ____

Applying Critical Thinking Skills to Test Questions

HELPFUL HINTS: Read all test questions carefully. Identify key words in the question that will guide you in answering the question. In these test questions the **key words** to consider are **"primarily," "correctly concludes,"** and **"most important."** Compare your rationale with the one in the test question.

1. The nurse clusters the client's objective and subjective signs and symptoms primarily to
   (a.) identify the nursing diagnosis.
   b. correlate with the medical diagnosis.
   c. validate the subjective complaints.
   d. work with at "risk for" diagnoses.

   Rationale: **(A) is the answer. Clustering the data helps the nurse to identify the defining characteristic that led to the formulation of a nursing diagnosis. Options (b) and (c) do not apply, and option (d) addresses only "risk for" diagnoses.**

2. The following nursing diagnosis is found on the client rand: Hip fracture r/t fall. In evaluating the written diagnosis, the nurse correctly concludes that the diagnosis
   a. is written appropriately.
   b. needs a modifier after the r/t statement.
   c. needs a modifier in the first part of the statement.
   (d) is written inappropriately.

   Rationale: **(D) is the answer. Hip fracture is a medical diagnosis. The nurse needs to identify the defining characteristics then select the appropriate nursing diagnosis. Options (a), (b), and (c) do not apply to this example.**

3. The nurse admits an elderly client with the medical diagnosis of dehydration. In developing the nursing diagnoses, it is most important for the nurse to
   a. establish nursing diagnoses that are based on the medical diagnosis.
   b. focus on nursing diagnoses that affect fluid balance.
   c. gather data to support actual nursing diagnoses.
   (d) include actual and risk for diagnoses.

   Rationale: **(D) is the answer. Nursing includes the development of actual nursing diagnoses as well as any risk for diagnoses in order to provide total, safe care to the client. Option (a) is not correct and options (b) and (c) do not include the monitoring of possible complications.**

ASSESSMENT OF THE ELDERLY PATIENT

List the **interventions** that would assist in communicating with an elderly patient who is experiencing hearing loss related to the aging process:

1. ______________________________
   ____
2. ______________________________
3. ______________________________
4. ______________________________
5. ______________________________
   ____

List the **interventions** that would assist an elderly patient who is experiencing vision problems related to the aging process:

1. ______________________________
2. ______________________________
   ____
3. ______________________________
   ____
4. ______________________________
5. ______________________________

Mark an **"X"** in the appropriate column that identifies the effects of aging on the following:

	Decreased	**Increased**
Sensory perception	☐	☐
Visual acuity	☐	☐
Gag reflex	☐	☐
Skin tissue elasticity	☐	☐
Body temperature	☐	☐
Cardiac output	☐	☐
RBC production	☐	☐
Plasma viscosity	☐	☐
Lung capacity	☐	☐
Residual urine	☐	☐

Case Study: The following information has been given to a group of students regarding the assessment of an elderly patient: Responds slowly but appropriately to all questions. Skin warm, dry, thin and flaky. Skin turgor >3 sec. Capillary refill >3 sec. Respirations short and shallow, lung sounds with bilateral crackles. 50% intake, states food is very bland. BM this morning moderate amount formed hard stool. Bilateral lower extremities with 1+ pitting edema. Toenails yellowish, thick. Vital signs T. 99° F - P. 84 - R.16 - B/P 160/80.

Pertinent Terminology	Definition
Arcus senilis	
Edema	
Pitting edema	
Kyphosis	
Presbycusis	
Presbyopia	
Turgor	

Use the information from the case study below to mark an **"X"** on the data that is representative of the normal effects of the aging process:

___ Responds slowly, but appropriately to all questions
___ Skin warm, dry, thin, and flaky
___ Skin turgor >3 sec; capillary refill >3 sec
___ Respirations short and shallow, lung sounds with bilateral crackles
___ 50% intake, states food is very bland
___ BM this morning formed hard stool
___ Bilateral lower extremities with 1+ pitting edema.
___ Toenails yellowish, thick
___ Vital signs T. 99° F - P. 84 - R. 16 - B/P 160/80

Interactive Activity: With a partner, use the information provided to **(1) underline** the assessment data that represent the **effects of the normal aging process** and **(2) select** the NANDA nursing diagnosis most appropriate for the situation:

Assessment Data	Nursing Diagnosis
Wife in to see patient, states that husband is confused this morning, does not know that he is in the hospital. Further patient assessment, PERRL, whitish ring noted around the margins of the iris, uses glasses. Mouth dry, wears upper dentures.	☐ Disturbed thought processes ☐ Impaired oral mucous membrane ☐ Acute confusion ☐ Impaired memory
Skin pale, translucent. Lower extremities thin, pedal pulses weak, palpable. States has loss of a small amount of urine when coughs. Shortness of breath, R 28, mouth breathing. Abdomen round, soft, nontender. Temp. 96.8° F.	☐ Functional urinary incontinence ☐ Hypothermia ☐ Ineffective tissue perfusion ☐ Ineffective breathing pattern
Transfers independently out of bed, complained of dizziness when coming to a standing position, gait slow. Anterior-posterior diameter of chest increased. Soft diet, intake 70%	☐ Impaired physical mobility ☐ Risk for injury ☐ Ineffective health maintenance ☐ Imbalanced nutrition: less than body requirements

CARING FOR THE SURGICAL PATIENT

List the **two major** types of anesthesia:

1. ____________________
2. ____________________

List the **types of regional anesthesia**:

1. ____________________
2. ____________________
3. ____________________
4. ____________________
5. ____________________

Identify in which of the perioperative phases (**preoperative**, **intraoperative**, **postoperative**) the following interventions would be started:

	Pre	Intra	Post
Use of incentive spirometer	☐	☐	☐
Coughing and deep breathing	☐	☐	☐
Splinting of surgical site	☐	☐	☐
Prepping surgical site	☐	☐	☐
Changing the surgical dressing	☐	☐	☐
Leg exercises	☐	☐	☐
Pain management	☐	☐	☐
Discharge instructions	☐	☐	☐

Case Study: A female patient is admitted for a total abdominal hysterectomy (TAH) this morning. She is 52 years old and is obese. Her past medical history indicates that she stopped smoking 5 years ago. Both parents are deceased. Mother died at the age of 88 and father died from a heart attack at the age of 62. The client's vital signs are: T. 97.8 - P. 76 - R. 18 - B/P 164/92. The following laboratory studies were done: CBC, PT, serum electrolytes of Na^+, K^+, serum FBS, BUN, and creatinine. The UA, chest x-ray report, and ECG report are in the chart.

Pertinent Terminology	Definition
General anesthesia	
Regional anesthesia	
Thrombophlebitis	
Atelectasis	
Paralytic ileus	
PCA	
Pneumatic compression device	

From the case study, **list** the factors that increase the patient's risk of postoperative complications:

* ____________________ * ____________________
* ____________________ * ____________________

Interactive Activity: With a partner, use the follow-up case study to **(1) identify** which medical order the nurse would do **first** and **(2) list the priority nursing interventions** the nurse would **independently perform** and provide a **rationale** for each intervention:

Follow-up case study: The patient returns from the postanesthesia room (PAR), sleepy but easily arousable. The physician writes the following postoperative orders:

NPO - May have sips of water in the AM
IV - Dextrose5/0.9 % Normal Saline infuse at 100 cc/hr
Ambulate this evening
VS q30 min for first hour, then q1h x2 hr, then q4h
Incentive spirometer q1h while awake
PCA - Morphine sulfate set at 1 mg/6 min (not to exceed 30 mg/4 hr)
Antiembolic stockings and pneumatic compression device to legs continuously
Indwelling urinary catheter to gravity - remove in AM

First Medical Orders to Implement	Rationale
1. ____________________	____________________

Priority Independent Nursing Interventions	Rationale
1. ____________________	____________________
2. ____________________	____________________
3. ____________________	____________________
4. ____________________	____________________
5. ____________________	____________________
6. ____________________	____________________
7. ____________________	____________________

Applying Critical Thinking Skills to Test Questions

INSTRUCTIONS: Circle the one best answer for each test question. Write your rationale for selecting the answer. To enhance your learning and test-taking skill, discuss your answer and rationale with a partner. The answer and the rationale can be found on the back of this page.

1. The client is transferred to the surgical unit from the postanesthesia room after having abdominal surgery. There is a J-P drainage device in place. Which of the following reported findings on transfer requires immediate follow-up?
   a. Abdominal dressing reinforced in the recovery room.
   b. R. 14, P. 86, B/P 126/90, lethargic, but responds to touch.
   c. Bowel sounds absent in all quadrants.
   d. J-P compressed with 10 cc reddish drainage.

   Rationale for your selection: ______________________________
   ____
   ____
   ____
   ____
   ____

2. Which of the following client statements is correct in describing the appropriate use of the incentive spirometer?
   a. "I will first inhale then blow into the mouthpiece."
   b. "I will put the mouthpiece in my mouth and blow into the mouthpiece."
   c. "I will put the mouthpiece in my mouth then inhale slowly."
   d. "I will put the mouthpiece in my mouth, inhale and hold for 5 seconds."

   Rationale for your selection: ______________________________
   ____
   ____
   ____
   ____
   ____

3. The nurse is preparing a client for emergency surgery. Before surgery, it is most important for the nurse to ensure that the
   a. pre-op checklist is completed.
   b. pre-op medications are documented.
   c. lab results are in the chart.
   d. surgical consent is signed.

   Rationale for your selection: ______________________________
   ____
   ____
   ____
   ____
   ____

Applying Critical Thinking Skills to Test Questions

HELPFUL HINTS: Read all test questions carefully. Identify key words in the question that will guide you in answering the question. In these test questions the **key words** to consider are **"immediate," "correct,"** and **"most important."** Compare your rationale with the one in the test question.

1. The client is transferred to the surgical unit from the postanesthesia room after having abdominal surgery. There is a J-P drainage device in place. Which of the following reported findings upon transfer requires immediate follow-up?
   (a.) Abdominal dressing reinforced in the recovery room.
   b. R. 14, P. 86, B/P 126/90, lethargic, but responds to touch.
   c. Bowel sounds absent in all quadrants.
   d. J-P compressed with 10 cc reddish drainage.

   Rationale: **(A) is the answer. Reinforcement of the surgical dressing indicates excessive drainage; this should be carefully monitored. Option (b) indicates vital signs WNL, and options (c) and (d) are expected findings for a client who had abdominal surgery.**

2. Which of the following client statements is correct in describing the appropriate use of the incentive spirometer?
   a. "I will first inhale then blow into the mouthpiece."
   b. "I will put the mouthpiece in my mouth and blow into the mouthpiece."
   (c.) "I will put the mouthpiece in my mouth then inhale slowly."
   d. "I will put the mouthpiece in my mouth, inhale and hold for 5 seconds."

   Rationale: **(C) is the answer – This describes the procedure appropriately. Options (a) and (b) do not describe the procedure correctly, and option (d) is partially correct but the client does not need to hold for 5 seconds.**

3. The nurse is preparing a client for emergency surgery. Before surgery, it is most important for the nurse to ensure that the
   a. pre-op checklist is completed.
   b. pre-op medications are documented.
   c. lab results are in the chart.
   (d.) surgical consent is signed.

   Rationale: **(D) is the answer. Although the physician is responsible for obtaining the client's signature, it is most important for the nurse to ensure that it has been signed. Options (a), (b), and (c) are important but are not the most important.**

WOUND ASSESSMENT

List the **types of wounds**:

1. ______________________
2. ______________________

List the **types of wound drainage** systems:

1. ______________________
2. ______________________
3. ______________________

Match the **wound classifications and wound drainage terminology** with the appropriate description or characteristics:

1. Laceration	___	Thin, clear watery secretion
2. Contusion	___	Containing pus
3. Penetrating	___	Open cut made with a knife/scalpel
4. Abrasion	___	Containing RBCs
5. Incision	___	Irregular wound tear; jagged edges
6. Serosangineous	___	Entering into the tissues/body cavity
7. Serous	___	Closed wound; with pain, swelling, and discoloration
8. Sangineous	___	Red, watery secretion
9. Purulent	___	A scraping away of the skin surface

Case Study: Mr. J, 26 years old, received a stab wound to his abdomen and was taken to the emergency room. He underwent emergency surgery. He has an IV, nasogastric tube to continuous low wall suction, and one Jackson-Pratt on the right upper quadrant and another on the left lower quadrant of the abdomen. He has a closed abdominal wound and the dressing is clean and dry as he is taken to he surgical unit at 0800.

Pertinent Terminology	Definition
Primary intention	
Tertiary intention	
Secondary intention	
Granulation tissue	
Inflammatory phase	
Proliferation phase	
Maturation phase	
Dehiscence	
Evisceration	

Use the case study to **check off (✓)** all the factors that apply to Mr. J:

- ☐ High risk for infection
- ☐ Healing by secondary intention
- ☐ J-P will aid in the healing process
- ☐ Post-op pain should initially increase
- ☐ J-P drainage should progressively decrease
- ☐ Slight redness around incision first day

Three hours after arriving on the surgical unit, the nurse took the vital signs and noted that Mr. J's surgical dressing has two abd pads and the dressing is currently saturated with sangineous drainage. The nurse lightly palpated the abdomen.

Abdominal Surgical Dressing

1100

Implement the appropriate nursing interventions on the abdominal surgical dressing:

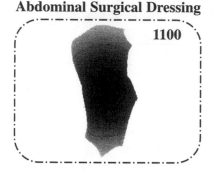

✗ **Select** the nurse's documentation that demonstrates appropriate assessment:

___ Abdominal dressing c̄ large amount of red drainage, abdomen tender, T 100.4° F

___ Abdominal dressing covered c̄ pink reddish drainage, abdomen tender, no bowel sounds, P. 88 - B/P 136/86.

___ Abdominal dressing saturated c̄ red drainage, abdomen tender, reinforced, P. 88 - B/P 136/86.

Interactive Activity: With a partner, use the **statements** below to **(1) check (✓) whether the statement is correct or incorrect and (2) provide a rationale for your selection.**

	Statements	Correct/Incorrect	Rationale
1.	Wound drainage devices need to be emptied once a shift.	☐ Correct ☐ Incorrect	____________ ____________
2.	Wound drainage devices need to be compressed to function.	☐ Correct ☐ Incorrect	____________ ____________
3.	Assessment of the wound should be done once a day.	☐ Correct ☐ Incorrect	____________ ____________
4.	Wound description does not need to include wound measurement.	☐ Correct ☐ Incorrect	____________ ____________
5.	Wound evisceration requires the application of sterile dry gauze.	☐ Correct ☐ Incorrect	____________ ____________

Applying Critical Thinking Skills to Test Questions

INSTRUCTIONS: Circle the one best answer for each test question. Write your rationale for selecting the answer. To enhance your learning and test-taking skill, discuss your answer and rationale with a partner. The answer and the rationale can be found on the back of this page.

1. An elderly client is being discharged after abdominal surgery. The staples were removed on the third day after surgery and a gauze dressing was applied. The client tells the nurse that as he was standing up he heard a pop coming from his abdomen. Which nursing intervention is of priority?
   a. Fully assess the neurologic status of the client.
   b. Auscultate the bowel sounds.
   c. Assess the surgical site.
   d. Palpate the abdomen.

   Rationale for your selection: ____________________

2. On the second day after surgery, the nurse assesses a surgical wound and documents the following, "Surgical incision with stitches intact, erythema noted on surrounding skin around surgical incision, edges well approximated." Based on this documentation, the nurse most accurately assessed that the surgical wound
   a. is healing without complications.
   b. is beginning to show signs of complications.
   c. needs to be assessed by the doctor.
   d. will take longer to heal.

   Rationale for your selection: ____________________

3. The physician orders the following dressing changes for an elderly client who has an open wound on the sacrum: "Apply hydrocolloid dressing on the wound. Change dressing every 3 days." The primary purpose of the dressing is to
   a. enhance healing by primary intention.
   b. absorb wound drainage.
   c. provide moisture to the area.
   d. protect the wound from additional pressure.

   Rationale for your selection: ____________________

Applying Critical Thinking Skills to Test Questions

HELPFUL HINTS: Read all test questions carefully. Identify key words in the question that will guide you in answering the question. In these test questions the **key words** to consider are **"priority," "most accurately,"** and **"primary purpose."** Compare your rationale with the one found for each question.

1. An elderly client is being discharged after abdominal surgery. The staples were removed on the third day after surgery and a gauze dressing was applied. The client tells the nurse that as he was standing up he heard a pop coming from his abdomen. Which nursing intervention is of priority?
   a. Fully assess the neurologic status of the client.
   b. Auscultate the bowel sounds.
   (c.) Assess the surgical site.
   d. Palpate the abdomen.

   Rationale: **(C) is the answer. Wound dehiscence is a possible complication. Clients may not have any pain. With option (a) not enough data are present to suggest that a full neurologic assessment is warranted and options (b) and (d) should be done after inspection.**

2. On the second day after surgery, the nurse assesses a surgical wound and documents the following, "Surgical incision with stitches intact, erythema noted on surrounding skin around surgical incision, edges well approximated." Based on this documentation, the nurse most accurately assessed that the surgical wound
   (a.) is healing without complications.
   b. is beginning to show signs of complications.
   c. needs to be assessed by the doctor.
   d. will take longer to heal.

   Rationale: **(A) is the answer. Documentation describes the normal healing process of a second postoperative day surgical wound. Options (b), (c), and (d) are not appropriate at this time.**

3. The physician orders the following dressing changes for an elderly client who has an open wound on the sacrum: "Apply hydrocolloid dressing on the wound. Change dressing every 3 days." The primary purpose of the dressing is to
   a. enhance healing by primary intention.
   (b.) absorb wound drainage.
   c. provide moisture to the area.
   d. protect the wound from additional pressure.

   Rationale: **(B) is the answer. Hydrocolloid dressings help to remove exudates from a wound. Option (a) is incorrect since the wound will heal by secondary intention; options (c) and (d) are not the primary purpose for applying this dressing.**

THE PATIENT WITH FLUID AND ELECTROLYTE IMBALANCE

List the **adult normal values** for the following electrolytes:

1. Sodium (Na^+) = ______________
2. Potassium (K^+) = ______________
3. Chloride (Cl^-) = ______________
4. Calcium (Ca^{2+}) = ______________
5. Phosphate (PO_4^-) = ______________
6. Magnesium (Mg^{2+}) = ______________

Write in the appropriate medical terminology for the serum laboratory values below:

Mg^{2+} 3.5 mg/dl = ______________

K^+ 2.5 mEq/L = ______________

Cl^- 90 mEq/L = ______________

Na^+ 132 mEq/L = ______________

Ca^{2+} 8.5 mg/dl = ______________

PO_4^- 5.1 mg/dl = ______________

Case Study: A 36-year-old client was admitted with gastroenteritis. He has been vomiting and having severe diarrhea for 2 days. He is very weak. The current laboratory results are: Na^+ 128 mEq/L, K^+ 2.8 mEq/L, Cl^- 90 mEq/L. The physician orders: IV of 0.9% NS at 100 cc/hr, NPO and I & O.

Pertinent Terminology	Definition
Sodium (Na^+)	
Potassium (K^+)	
Chloride (Cl^-)	
Calcium (Ca^{2+})	
Phosphate (PO_4^-)	
Magnesium (Mg^{2+})	
Third space syndrome	
Edema	
Pitting edema	

From the case study, identify the abnormal laboratory results. List the **major clinical signs or symptoms** that you would assess with each abnormal value:

* ________________ = ____
____
____

* ________________ = ____

* ________________ = ____
____
____

☞ **Follow-up case study:** The client's vomiting and diarrhea has begun to subside in the evening and the MD has ordered a clear liquid diet. The client's **24-hour I & O** for the day is charted below:

24-Hour Intake/Output Record

Intake			Output		
IV	=	2400	Emesis	=	950
Oral	=	120	Diarrhea	=	900
			Urine	=	750
		2520 cc			2600 cc

☞ Based on the case study and Intake and Output Record **select** the most appropriate **NANDA Nursing Diagnoses** for the client:

___ Excess fluid volume
___ Diarrhea
___ Imbalanced nutrition: Less than body requirements
___ Deficient fluid volume
___ Impaired skin integrity
___ Risk for injury

Interactive Activity: With a partner, read the case study below and write a rationale for each of the nursing interventions listed:

Case Study	Nursing Interventions	Rationale
Ms. M was admitted with heart failure. The nursing diagnosis of "Fluid volume excess r/t noncompliance to dietary Na^+ restriction" is listed in her NCP. Digoxin 0.25 mg qd po, Furosemide 40 mg qd po, and K-dur 10 mEq po tid are her medications.	➢ Weigh daily	________________
	➢ Monitor I & O	________________
	➢ Take apical pulse	________________
	➢ Assess skin	________________
	➢ Assess lungs	________________
	➢ ✓ Neck veins	________________

GASTROINTESTINAL TRACT

List the structures in the gastrointestinal tract involved with the digestion and absorption of food:

1. ______________________
2. ______________________
3. ______________________
4. ______________________
5. ______________________

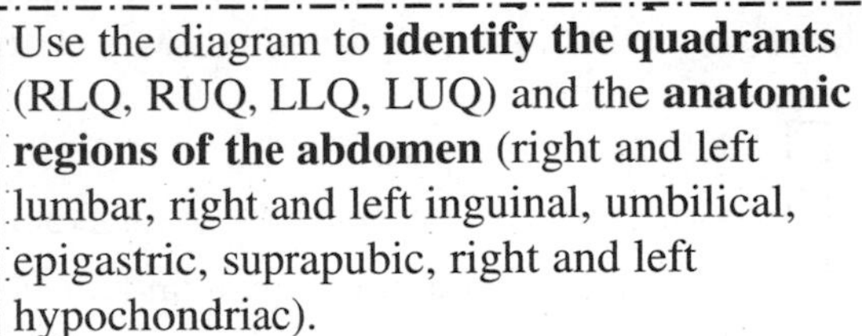

Use the diagram to **identify the quadrants** (RLQ, RUQ, LLQ, LUQ) and the **anatomic regions of the abdomen** (right and left lumbar, right and left inguinal, umbilical, epigastric, suprapubic, right and left hypochondriac).

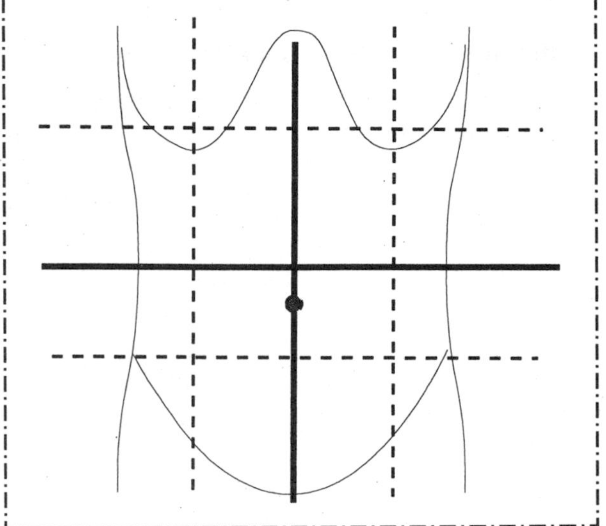

Modified from Black JM, Hawks JH, Keene AM: *Medical-surgical nursing: clinical management for positive outcomes*, ed 6, Philadelphia, 2001, WB Saunders.

Case Study: Mrs. T is a 55-year-old woman who was admitted to the hospital with complaints of diarrhea for the past 10 days. She states that she has abdominal cramping and at times passes bloody stools. She is scheduled for a colonoscopy at 10:00 AM today.

Pertinent Terminology	Definition
Duodenum	
Jejunum	
Ileum	
Cecum	
Colon	
Rectum	
Polyp	

Use the case study to (✓) **check off all the nursing interventions and physician's orders** that you would associate with the preparation of Mrs. T for the colonoscopy procedure.

- ☐ NPO for procedure
- ☐ GoLytely will be given for stool evacuation
- ☐ Monitor for abdominal pain and bleeding postprocedure
- ☐ Consent is necessary
- ☐ May have a clear liquid breakfast
- ☐ Requires general anesthesia

Match the gastrointestinal diagnostic tests with the appropriate definitions:

Diagnostic tests		Definitions
1. Colonoscopy	___	Visualization of the rectum and sigmoid
2. Endoscopy	___	Visualization from anus to cecum
3. Sigmoidoscopy	___	Visualization of esophagus, stomach, and small bowel
4. Barium swallow	___	Visualization of interior organs and structures using a fiberoptic instrument

Interactive Activity: With a partner, use the diagram to

1. Identify the segments of the large intestine.
2. Follow the path of the colonoscopy procedure.
3. Identify the consistency of the stool as it moves through the intestinal tract (mushy, semi-liquid, and solid).

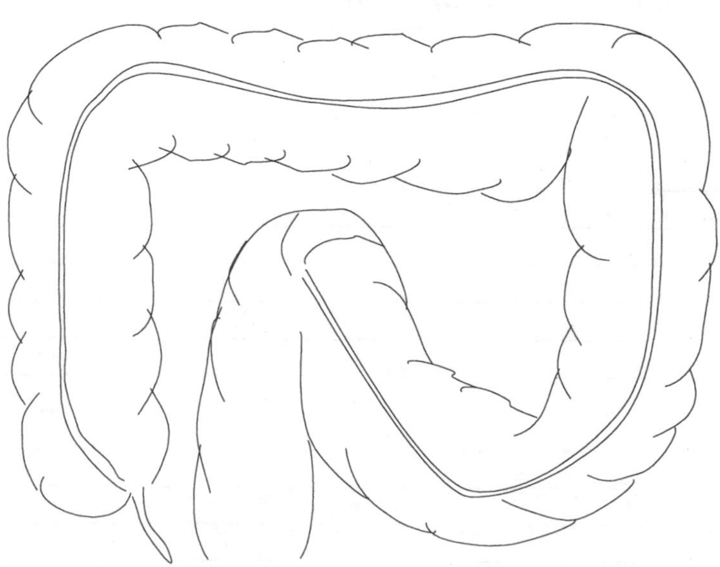

Applying Critical Thinking Skills to Test Questions

INSTRUCTIONS: Circle the one best answer for each test question. Write your rationale for selecting the answer. To enhance your learning and test-taking skill, discuss your answer and rationale with a partner. The answer and the rationale can be found on the back of this page.

1. The client is scheduled for an UGI endoscopy. Which statement is correct in providing the client with information about this endoscopic procedure?
   a. "A tube will be passed from your nose into your stomach."
   b. "The tube is small, is very flexible, and has a light at the end."
   c. "The tube has a light that will allow the doctor to see your intestines."
   d. "A tube will be passed from your mouth and into your stomach."

   Rationale for your selection: ______________________________

2. The day after having a barium enema as an outpatient, the client calls the clinic nurse to express concern because the stools are white in color. Which statement made by the nurse is most helpful?
   a. "Don't worry, this is normal after a barium enema."
   b. "This is expected, be sure to drink plenty of fluids."
   c. "The stool color should return after 1 to 2 days."
   d. "This is expected, call back if your stools are still white after 5 days."

   Rationale for your selection: ______________________________

3. The nurse is taking care of a 76-year-old client who is having an upper GI series this morning. After the completion of the procedure, the nurse should initially
   a. see if a laxative is ordered for the client.
   b. assess the bowel sounds.
   c. take the vital signs.
   d. observe for intestinal obstruction.

   Rationale for your selection: ______________________________

Applying Critical Thinking Skills to Test Questions

HELPFUL HINTS: Read all test questions carefully. Identify key words in the question that will guide you in answering the question. In these test questions the **key words** to consider are **"correct," "most helpful,"** and **"initially."** Compare your rationale with the one in the test question.

1. The client is scheduled for an UGI endoscopy. Which statement is correct in providing the client with information about this endoscopic procedure?
   a. "A tube will be passed from your nose into your stomach."
   b. "The tube is small, is very flexible, and has a light at the end."
   c. "The tube has a light that will allow the doctor to see your intestines."
   (d.) "A tube will be passed from your mouth and into your stomach."

   Rationale: **(D) is the answer. This is a beginning statement that informs the client as to how the procedure will be carried out. Options (a), (b), and (c) do not provide accurate information about the procedure.**

2. The day after having a barium enema as an outpatient, the client calls the clinic nurse to express concern because the stools are white in color. Which statement made by the nurse is most helpful?
   a. "Don't worry, this is normal after a barium enema."
   (b.) "This is expected, be sure to drink plenty of fluids."
   c. "The stool color should return after 1 to 2 days."
   d. "This is expected, call back if your stools are still white after 5 days."

   Rationale: **(B) is the answer. It is important to reassure the client and to provide instructions that help minimize complications. Barium impaction is a concern after a barium enema. Options (a), (c), and (d) do not provide enough information.**

3. The nurse is taking care of a 76-year-old client who is having an upper GI series this morning. After the completion of the procedure, the nurse should initially
   (a.) see if a laxative is ordered for the client.
   b. assess the bowel sounds.
   c. take the vital signs.
   d. observe for intestinal obstruction.

   Rationale: **(A) is the answer. To prevent the complication of fecal impaction after an UGI series (barium swallow) a laxative is usually given following the procedure. Options (b) and (c) are good interventions, but the situation does not address the need for these interventions; option (d) does not focus on the initial intervention.**

DIABETES MELLITUS

List the classic **signs and symptoms** of **diabetes mellitus**:

» ______________________

» ______________________

» ______________________

List other signs and symptoms associated with hyperglycemia:

» ______________________

» ______________________

» ______________________

» ______________________

» ______________________

» ______________________

» ______________________

Fill in the **circles** that identify the **signs and symptoms** associated with **hypoglycemia**.

- O Polyuria
- O Shakiness
- O Tremor
- O Irritability
- O Glucosuria
- O Polydipsia
- O Sweating
- O Confusion
- O Dizziness
- O Blurred vision
- O Hunger
- O Slurred speech
- O Paresthesia
- O Tachycardia

Case Study: A 20-year-old woman makes an appointment with her doctor with complaints of feeling fatigued and lethargic for several days. She states that she has noticed that she has lost 15 lb. She tells the doctor that she does not understand why she has lost so much weight since she has been eating a lot. The doctor asks if she voids more than usual. Marty says that she does but that she thinks it is because of all the water that she is drinking all day.

Pertinent Terminology	Definition
Diabetes mellitus (DM)	
Type 1 diabetes	
Type 2 diabetes	
Insulin resistance	
Insulin	
Counterregulatory hormones	
Oral hypoglycemics agents	

The doctor orders a fasting blood sugar (FBS) test and an FBS with a 2 hr postprandial test for the patient. The following results are noted in her clinic chart. **Write in** the normal laboratory value for the test in the column provided.

Test	Results	Normal laboratory values
FBS	160 mg/dl	______________
2 hr PP	225 mg/dl	______________

Marty is informed that she has type 1 diabetes mellitus. **Fill in** the circles that correlate with the diagnosis and treatment of type 1 diabetes mellitus.

- O Oral hypoglycemics will be ordered
- O Exercise is part of the treatment plan
- O Will need to monitor for signs and symptoms of hypoglycemia
- O Insulin will be required every day
- O Will require blood glucose testing
- O Beta cells are producing insulin
- O Will need to monitor for signs and symptoms of hyperglycemia
- O Will not need insulin if follows diet

Interactive Activity: With a partner, use the **Key Points Box** and the **Follow-up case study** to **identify the response(s)** that should be included in responding to each question. **Write** the letter in the **Responses** section to identify the responses you have selected.

Key Points Box

A. "Usually ½ hr to 1 hr before breakfast"
B. "Insulin needs may change over time"
C. "Check blood sugar level"
D. "Always carry oral glucose tablets"
E. "Destroyed by the gastric enzymes"
F. "No"
G. "Drink orange, apple or grape juice"
H. "Know the signs and symptoms of hypoglycemia"

Follow-up case study: The patient is started on Humulin NPH insulin 10 U qAM and NPH 5 U qPM. She is taught how to do self-monitoring blood glucose checks (SMBG) qid.

	Responses
1. "When is the best time to administer the AM insulin?"	________
2. "If I forget the PM dose of insulin, can I double the dose in the morning?"	________
3. "What should I do if I begin to get shaky and dizzy?"	________
4. "How do I prepare for a hypoglycemic reaction?"	________

Applying Critical Thinking Skills to Test Questions

INSTRUCTIONS: Circle the one best answer for each test question. Write your rationale for selecting the answer. To enhance your learning and test-taking skill, discuss your answer and rationale with a partner. The answer and the rationale can be found on the back of this page.

1. A client is diagnosed with diabetes mellitus type 1. In teaching the client about diabetes mellitus type 1, it is most important for the client to
   a. know how to use hypoglycemic agents to control the diabetes.
   b. understand that insulin injections will be required daily.
   c. randomly check finger stick blood glucose throughout the day.
   d. decrease physical activity.

   Rationale for your selection: ____

   ____
   ____
   ____
   ____
   ____

2. The nurse learns in morning report that the 0700 fasting blood glucose of a client was 74 mg/dl. Which of the following morning assessment findings is of priority?
   a. Abdominal wound dressing with moderate dried red drainage.
   b. Complaining of thirst and dried mouth.
   c. Output of 250 cc during the night shift.
   d. Diaphoresis noted while taking vital signs.

   Rationale for your selection: ____

   ____
   ____
   ____
   ____
   ____

3. The nurse is assigned to a client who has just been diagnosed with diabetes mellitus type 1. Which of the following assessment findings is most consistent with this diagnosis?
   a. FBS 110 mg/dl, hypertension, decreased urinary output
   b. Random BS >140 mg/dl, obese, limited physical activity
   c. Weight loss, episodes of shakiness and diaphoresis
   d. Frequent urination, hunger, and excessive fluid intake

   Rationale for your selection: ____

   ____
   ____
   ____
   ____
   ____

Applying Critical Thinking Skills to Test Questions

HELPFUL HINTS: Read all test questions carefully. Identify key words in the question that will guide you in answering the question. In these test questions the **key words** to consider are **"most important," "priority,"** and **"most consistent."** Compare your rationale with the one in the test question.

1. A client is diagnosed with diabetes mellitus type 1. In teaching the client about diabetes mellitus type 1, it is most important for the client to
   a. know how to use hypoglycemic agents to control the diabetes.
   (b.) understand that insulin injections will be required daily.
   c. randomly check finger stick blood glucose throughout the day.
   d. decrease physical activity.

   Rationale: **(B) is the answer. With diabetes mellitus type 1 the beta cells have stopped functioning and the use of exogenous insulin administration is required. Option (a) is not appropriate for type 1 diabetes mellitus since hypoglycemic agents are used for type 2 DM. Option (c)—blood glucose is monitored at specific times for control and with (d) exercise is recommended.**

2. The nurse learns in morning report that the 0700 fasting blood glucose of a client was 74 mg/dl. Which of the following morning assessment findings is of priority?
   a. Abdominal wound dressing with moderate dried red drainage.
   b. Complaining of thirst and dried mouth.
   c. Output of 250 cc during the night shift.
   (d.) Diaphoresis noted while taking vital signs.

   Rationale: **(D) is the answer. Diaphoresis is a sign associated with hypoglycemia and should be assessed further. Also, the morning blood sugar was toward the lower limit of normal. Options (a) and (c) are WNL, and option (b) is important but not a priority.**

3. The nurse is assigned to a client who has just been diagnosed with diabetes mellitus type 1. Which of the following assessment findings is most consistent with this diagnosis?
   a. FBS 110 mg/dl, hypertension, decreased urinary output
   b. Random BS > 140 mg/dl, obese, limited physical activity
   c. Weight loss, episodes of shakiness and diaphoresis
   (d) Frequent urination, hunger, and excessive fluid intake

   Rationale: **(D) is the answer. The classic signs and symptoms associated with diabetes mellitus type 1 are polyuria, polydipsia, and polyphagia. Options (a), (b), and (c) are not the most consistent with the diagnosis.**

COMPLICATIONS OF DIABETES MELLITUS

List the **causes** that precipitate **hypoglycemic reactions**:

» ______________________________

» ______________________________

» ______________________________

» ______________________________

» ______________________________

List the **causes** that precipitate the development of **diabetic ketoacidosis**:

» ______________________________

» ______________________________

» ______________________________

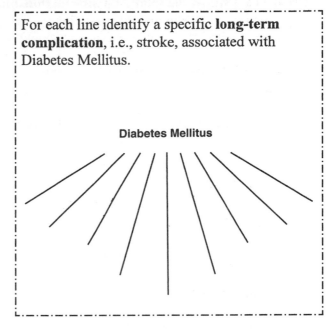

For each line identify a specific **long-term complication**, i.e., stroke, associated with Diabetes Mellitus.

Diabetes Mellitus

Case Study: Mr. E, 56 years old, has been a diabetic for 25 years. He is admitted to the hospital after experiencing a cerebral vascular accident (CVA). His wife says that her husband monitors his blood glucose daily and administers his own insulin. However, she tells the nurse that he does not always stick to his diet. She wonders whether this may have contributed to the CVA. Mr. E has an order for NPH insulin 36 U qAM and NPH 17 U qPM with blood glucose finger sticks ac and HS. He is started on a sliding scale.

Pertinent Terminology	Definition
Lipoatrophy	
Lipohypertrophy	
Impaired glucose tolerance	
Somogyi effect	
Dawn phenomenon	
Diabetic ketoacidosis (DKA)	
Hyperglycemic hyperosmolar nonketotic coma (HHNK)	

Use the **case study, the follow-up information, and the nursing interventions below** to plan out Mr. E's morning care in the order of **priority**. Place a number, beginning with #1, in each box to indicate the sequence of the nursing care that should be delivered by the nurse.

Follow-up information: The AM blood glucose finger stick and insulin are to be done by the morning shift. Mr. E is started on a diet containing semithick liquids.

Nursing Interventions	Rationale
☐ Perform a body systems assessment	______
☐ Perform a finger stick	______
☐ Take the AM vital signs	______
☐ Administer morning insulin	______
☐ Perform morning care	______
☐ Provide information regarding the complications of diabetes	______
☐ Assist with breakfast	______

Place a check (✔) next to the statements that are correct regarding the use of a sliding scale.

___ Only regular insulin is used

___ Dosage based on ac BS levels

___ May be combined with other insulins

___ Used for patients with DM type 1

___ Used for patients with DM type 2

___ Used during periods of illness

Interactive Activity: The following nursing diagnosis is found on Mr. E's nursing care plan. With a partner, **write the three most important nursing interventions for the nursing diagnosis**.

Nursing Diagnosis	Nursing Interventions
Risk for aspiration r/t impaired swallowing secondary to CVA	1. ______ 2. ______ 3. ______

Applying Critical Thinking Skills to Test Questions

INSTRUCTIONS: Circle the one best answer for each test question. Write your rationale for selecting the answer. To enhance your learning and test-taking skill, discuss your answer and rationale with a partner. The answer and the rationale can be found on the back of this page.

1. The nurse notes that the assigned client has an A/V fistula on the right arm and is scheduled for hemodialysis this morning. In delegating the care of the client, it is most important for the nurse to
   a. inform the nursing assistant to give the bath after the hemodialysis.
   b. direct that all morning care is done before hemodialysis.
   c. instruct that the blood pressure be taken on the left arm.
   d. ask that the client be weighed first.

   Rationale for your selection: ____
   ____
   ____
   ____
   ____
   ____

2. The nurse is admitting a client with uncontrolled diabetes mellitus. The client has left- sided hemiparesis from a previous cerebral vascular accident. The client's admitting blood glucose was 325 mg/dl. Which of the following nursing diagnosis is of priority?
   a. Rick for fluid volume deficit
   b. Fluid volume overload
   c. Ineffective tissue perfusion
   d. Noncompliance

   Rationale for your selection: ____
   ____
   ____
   ____
   ____
   ____

3. The nurse is taking care of a client who has diabetes mellitus type 1. The client tells the nurse that he is beginning to feel symptoms of hypoglycemia. Which action by the nurse is of priority?
   a. Have the client drink a glass of orange juice.
   b. Monitor for signs of hypoglycemia.
   c. Take the pulse, respirations, and blood pressure.
   d. Have the laboratory perform a blood glucose test stat.

   Rationale for your selection: ____
   ____
   ____
   ____
   ____
   ____

Applying Critical Thinking Skills to Test Questions

HELPFUL HINTS: Read all test questions carefully. Identify key words in the question that will guide you in answering the question. In these test questions the **key words** to consider are **"most important"** and **"priority."** Compare your rationale with the one in the test question.

1. The nurse notes that the assigned client has an A/V fistula on the right arm and is scheduled for hemodialysis this morning. In delegating the care of the client, it is most important for the nurse to
   a. inform the nursing assistant to give the bath after the hemodialysis.
   b. direct that all morning care is done before hemodialysis.
   (c.) instruct that the blood pressure be taken on the left arm.
   d. ask that the client be weighed first.

   Rationale: **(C) is the answer. It is most important to ensure the patency of the A/V fistula and prevent vascular complications that can occur with applied pressure from the B/P cuff. Options (a) and (b) can be done anytime, and although option (d) is important, it is not the most important based on this situation.**

2. The nurse is admitting a client with uncontrolled diabetes mellitus. The client has left- sided hemiparesis from a previous cerebral vascular accident. The client's admitting blood glucose was 325 mg/dl. Which of the following nursing diagnosis is of priority?
   (a.) Rick for fluid volume deficit
   b. Fluid volume overload
   c. Ineffective tissue perfusion
   d. Noncompliance

   Rationale: **(A) is the answer. The body will attempt to excrete the excessive glucose and will also excrete water and electrolytes predisposing the client to dehydration. Options (b), (c), and (d) are important, but they are not priorities during the acute phase.**

3. The nurse is taking care of a client who has diabetes mellitus type 1. The client tells the nurse that he is beginning to feel symptoms of hypoglycemia. Which action by the nurse is of priority?
   (a.) Have the client drink a glass of orange juice.
   b. Monitor for signs of hypoglycemia.
   c. Take the pulse, respirations, and blood pressure.
   d. Have the laboratory perform a blood glucose test stat.

   Rationale: **(A) is the answer. The hypoglycemic effects can occur rapidly. It is always better to treat hypoglycemia in the early stages then to allow for central nervous system involvement. Options (b), (c), and (d) do not focus on the immediate treatment.**

INSULIN THERAPY

List the **onset**, **peak**, and **duration** of the following insulins:

Rapid acting:

Onset ______________________
Peak ______________________
Duration ______________________

Short acting:

Onset ______________________
Peak ______________________
Duration ______________________

Intermediate acting:

Onset ______________________
Peak ______________________
Duration ______________________

Long acting:

Onset ______________________
Peak ______________________
Duration ______________________

Using the boxes on the left column write **(R)** if the insulin is rapid acting, **(S)** if the insulin is short acting, **(I)** if the insulin is intermediate acting, and **(L)** if the insulin is long acting.

☐	NPH	☐
☐	Lantus	☐
☐	Ultralente	☐
☐	Lente	☐
☐	Humulin R	☐
☐	Humulin N	☐
☐	Humalog-Lispro	☐
☐	Novolog	☐

Place an **"X"** on column to the right to identify the insulin that may be given **IV**.

Case Study: Marty, 22 years old, has been on Humulin NPH insulin since her diagnosis of DM Type 1 two years ago. Marty administers 12 Units NPH with 5 Units Regular insulin q.AM and 4 Units NPH q.PM. She monitors her blood sugar q.i.d. ac and HS, and routinely administers the AM insulin dose at 0700 and the PM dose at 1700. Marty maintains a daily chart of her blood sugar results.

Pertinent Terminology	Definition
Glucagon	
Glycogenolysis	
Gluconeogenesis	
Glycosylated hemoglobin	
Glycosylated albumin	
Oral glucose tolerance test	
Hypoglycemia	

From the case study, plot out Marty's morning dose of NPH and Regular insulin on the **Insulin Progression Graph**. Begin with the **onset (O)** followed by identifying the **peak of action (P)** of the insulin and the **duration (D)**.

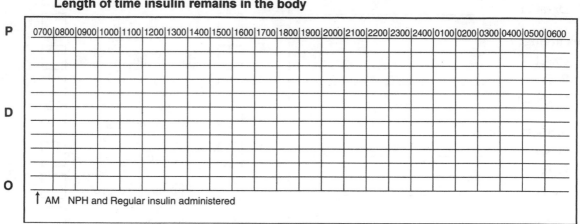

Insulin Progression Graph
Onset ➔ Peak ➔ Duration

Length of time insulin remains in the body

P

0700	0800	0900	1000	1100	1200	1300	1400	1500	1600	1700	1800	1900	2000	2100	2200	2300	2400	0100	0200	0300	0400	0500	0600

D

O

↑ AM NPH and Regular insulin administered

Marty eats a full breakfast 0800 but is unable to eat lunch. Use the **Insulin Progressive Graph** to indicate the time Marty would most likely experience a **hypoglycemic episode.** ______________

Select (✓) the most appropriate **snack** for Marty to eat if she experiences a hypoglycemic reaction at 1600 and has a fingerstick blood glucose of 64 mg/dl.

____ 6 saltine crackers
____ 4 oz apple juice
____ 8 oz diet soda

Interactive Activity: With a partner, **underline** the **correct word** in each statement as it relates to the sentence and **provide a rationale** for your selection.

1. For the patient with DM type 1, moderate exercise may have **hyperglycemic** or **hypoglycemic** effects.

   Rationale: ____

   ____

2. A patient with DM type 1 performs a finger stick before exercising and the blood glucose results are 92 mg/dl. The patient should eat a snack **before** or **immediately after** exercising.

   Rationale: ____

   ____

   ____

3. Alcohol consumption puts the patient with DM type 1 at risk for **hypoglycemia - hyperglycemia**.

   Rationale: ____

   ____

Applying Critical Thinking Skills to Test Questions

INSTRUCTIONS: Circle the one best answer for each test question. Write your rationale for selecting the answer. To enhance your learning and test-taking skill, discuss your answer and rationale with a partner. The answer and the rationale can be found on the back of this page.

1. The nurse learns in report that the assigned client has a finger stick blood glucose result of 100 mg/dl at 0700. The client receives NPH insulin 15 U SC qAM. Based on the morning report, it is most appropriate for the nurse to
   a. hold the AM dose of insulin.
   b. administer the AM dose of insulin.
   c. call the doctor to report the blood glucose results.
   d. repeat the finger stick blood glucose test at 0800.

   Rationale for your selection: ______________________________

2. The doctor orders Lente insulin 23 U SC qAM. The nurse carries out this order correctly when the insulin
   a. dose is given after breakfast.
   b. dose is based on the finger stick blood glucose results.
   c. is given according to the hospital's qAM schedule.
   d. is administered before breakfast.

   Rationale for your selection: ______________________________

3. A client with DM type 1 had a sliding scale using regular insulin listed on the patient care rand. Based on this finding, it is most important for the nurse to
   a. administer the regular insulin based on the FBS.
   b. monitor the client's urine for ketones before meals.
   c. obtain finger stick blood glucose test before meals.
   d. check the finger stick blood glucose qid.

   Rationale for your selection: ______________________________

Applying Critical Thinking Skills to Test Questions

HELPFUL HINTS: Read all test questions carefully. Identify key words in the question that will guide you in answering the question. In these test questions the **key words** to consider are **"most appropriate," "correctly,"** and **"most important."** Compare your rationale with the one in the test question.

1. The nurse learns in report that the assigned client has a finger stick blood glucose result of 100 mg/dl at 0700. The client receives NPH insulin 15 U SC qAM. Based on the morning report, it is most appropriate for the nurse to
   a. hold the AM dose of insulin.
   (b) administer the AM dose of insulin.
   c. call the doctor to report the blood glucose results.
   d. repeat the finger stick blood glucose test at 0800.

   Rationale: **(B) is the answer. The finger stick blood glucose results are WNL. The nurse should administer the daily dose of insulin. Options (a), (c), and (d) are not appropriate interventions based on this situation.**

2. The doctor orders Lente insulin 23 U SC qAM. The nurse carries out this order correctly when the insulin
   a. dose is given after breakfast.
   b. dose is based on the finger stick blood glucose results.
   c. is given according to the hospital's qAM schedule.
   (d) is administered before breakfast.

   Rationale: **(D) is the answer. Although daily insulin is ordered qAM, the ordered dose is given before breakfast to correlate with the action of the insulin and food intake. Options (a) and (c) are similar and start after food intake. Option (b) is used mostly with regular insulin.**

3. A client with DM type 1 had a sliding scale using regular insulin listed on the patient care rand. Based on this finding, it is most important for the nurse to
   a. administer the regular insulin based on the FBS.
   b. monitor the client's urine for ketones before meals.
   (c.) obtain finger stick blood glucose test before meals.
   d. check the finger stick blood glucose qid.

   Rationale: **(C) is the answer. The sliding scale is used to administer regular insulin throughout the day based on finger stick blood glucose levels. Options (a), (b), and (d) do not correlate the purpose of the sliding scale, regular insulin, blood glucose, and food intake.**

SECTION TWO

Priority-Setting and Decision-Making Activities

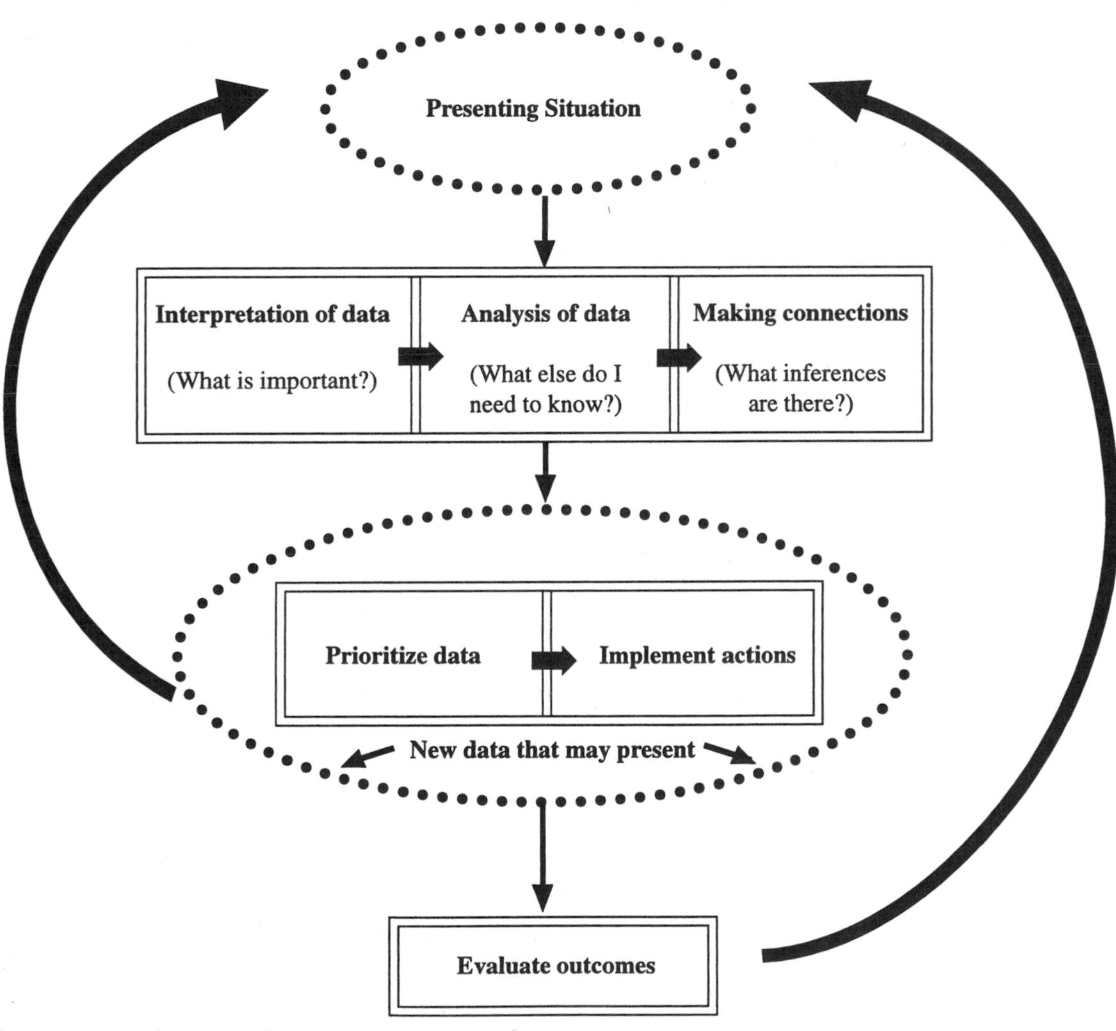

THE PATIENT UNDERGOING SURGERY

Mr. H, age 60, was admitted with persistent abdominal pain. He states he has had nausea and vomiting and has noticed a 10 lb weight loss within the last 2 months. He is diagnosed with gastric cancer and is scheduled for a subtotal gastrectomy in the morning. He has Demerol 75 mg with Phenergen 25 mg IM q3-4 hr prn pain and Mylanta 30 cc po q2h prn abdominal pain. Mr. H is very anxious after speaking with his physician and refuses to sign the surgical consent. He tells the nurse that he is having abdominal pain and "wants his pain shot right now." The nurse notes that it is just about 3 hours since his last pain medication.

Instructions: Prioritize the following **nursing interventions** as you, the nurse, would do them to initially take care of Mr. H. Write a number in the box to identify the order of your interventions (#1 = first intervention, #2 = second intervention, etc.) and state a **rationale** for each intervention.

INTERVENTIONS	PRIORITY #	RATIONALE
◆ Administer IM pain med.	☐	
◆ Sit and talk with patient	☐	
◆ Give Mylanta 30 cc	☐	
◆ Offer to call a family member	☐	
◆ Notify physician	☐	

KEY POINTS TO CONSIDER:

Mr. H does consent to have surgery and returns to the medical unit post-op. He has an IV of lactated Ringer's infusing at 125 cc/hr and you note the following:

1. P. 90 - R. 20 - B/P 130/76
2. He is alert and oriented and his skin is warm and dry
3. N/G tube draining brown-reddish drainage (300 cc in the last 4 hours)
4. Indwelling urinary catheter draining light yellow urine (700 cc in the last 4 hours)

✓✓✓ **Interactive activity:** With a partner, **do the following: (1) based on the current assessment, select** the **one nursing diagnosis** that is of priority at this time, **(2) provide a rationale** for your selection, and **(3) list three nursing interventions** that meet the needs of Mr. H:

All of the following nursing diagnoses may apply to Mr. H:

Risk for infection, Pain, Anxiety, Ineffective airway clearance, Fatigue, Impaired physical mobility, Imbalanced nutrition: less than body requirements, Deficient knowledge, Risk for deficient fluid volume, Fear.

Nursing Diagnosis	Rationale	Nursing Interventions
		1. **2.** **3.**

✓✓✓ Several hours after surgery you note that Mr. H is very restless and you assess:

R. 32 - P. 130 - B/P 108/70, N/G drainage 200 cc bright red drainage, skin cool, c/o pain

Instructions: Based on the situation, identify and write the **priority problem** in the box below. Then, starting with the small box labeled ***#1*** **prioritize** the **nursing interventions** for this situation and identify your plan for follow-up care for Mr. H.

NURSING INTERVENTIONS

A. Monitor P, R, B/P, & pulse oximetry
B. Document assessment/nursing care
C. Prepare for gastric lavage
D. Plan to start oxygen therapy
E. Stay with Mr. H
F. Notify physician

DECISION-MAKING DIAGRAM

New Action Plan

#1 #2 #3 #4 #5 #6

Priority Problem

NOTES ____________________

____

Applying Critical Thinking Skills to Test Questions

INSTRUCTIONS: Circle the one best answer for each test question. Write your rationale for selecting the answer. To enhance your learning and test-taking skill, discuss your answer and rationale with a partner. The answer and the rationale can be found on the back of this page.

1. The nurse assesses the following on a client who had a colon resection 5 days ago: A & O × 4, skin warm, abd distended nontender, bowel sounds present. Abd sutures approximated. States pain level 2. IV infusing at 75 cc/hr per pump. Fine crackles in the bilateral lower lung bases. In planning care, which nursing action is of priority?
   a. Take vital signs q4h
   b. Ambulate the client
   c. Assess lung sounds q4h
   d. Push oral fluids

   Rationale: ____

   ____

   ____

   ____

   ____

2. The nurse is caring for a client who has diabetes mellitus type 1 and is 2 days post-op abdominal surgery. The client takes clopidrogrel (Plavix) 75 mg po qd and aspirin 81 mg po qd. In preparing the administration of these drugs, it is most important for the nurse to first
   a. assess if the client is having mild pain.
   b. check the serum protime levels.
   c. monitor the blood pressure.
   d. ensure that the client has eaten.

   Rationale: ____

   ____

   ____

   ____

   ____

3. The nurse administers atropine gr 1/150 IM as ordered pre-op for surgery. Thirty minutes after administration, the client complains of a very dry mouth and has flushed, dry skin with an oral temperature of 99° F and a pulse rate of 104. The most appropriate nursing action is for the nurse to
   a. document the client's complaints.
   b. notify the physician.
   c. take the client's temperature in 1 hour.
   d. recognize that these are normal side effects of the drug.

   Rationale: ____

   ____

   ____

   ____

   ____

Applying Critical Thinking Skills to Test Questions

HELPFUL HINTS: Read all test questions carefully. Identify key words in the question that will guide you in answering the question. In these test questions the **key words** to consider are **"priority," "most important,"** and **"most appropriate."** Compare your rationale with the one in the test question.

1. The nurse assesses the following on a client who had a colon resection 5 days ago: A & O × 4, skin warm, abd distended nontender, bowel sounds present. Abd sutures approximated. States pain level 2. IV infusing at 75 cc/hr per pump. Fine crackles in the bilateral lower lung bases. In planning care, which nursing action is of priority?
   a. Take vital signs q4h
   (b) Ambulate the client
   c. Assess lung sounds q4h
   d. Push oral fluids

   Rationale: **(B) is the answer. Assessment data indicate the need to ambulate the client to ease abdominal distention and enhance respiration and movement of secretions. Options (a), (c), and (d) are important but do not help the client with the priority problems.**

2. The nurse is caring for a client who has diabetes mellitus type 1 and is 2 days post-op abdominal surgery. The client takes clopidrogrel (Plavix) 75 mg po qd and aspirin 81 mg po qd. In preparing the administration of these drugs, it is most important for the nurse to first
   a. assess if the client is having mild pain.
   (b.) check the serum protime levels.
   c. monitor the blood pressure.
   d. ensure that the client has eaten.

   Rationale: **(B) is the answer. Clopidrogrel and aspirin both have anticoagulation properties. Coagulation studies should be monitored throughout therapy. Options (a), (c), and (d) do not address the most important intervention related to this drug therapy.**

3. The nurse administers atropine gr 1/150 IM as ordered pre-op for surgery. Thirty minutes after administration, the client complains of a very dry mouth and has flushed, dry skin with an oral temperature of 99° F and a pulse rate of 104. The most appropriate nursing action is for the nurse to
   a. document the client's complaints.
   (b.) notify the physician.
   c. take the client's temperature in 1 hour.
   d. recognize that these are normal side effects of the drug.

   Rationale: **(B) is the answer. Atropine is a cholinergic blocking agent. The client is manifesting symptoms of adverse effects. Options (a) and (c) are not the most important. There is a narrow margin between the side effects and the adverse effects of the drug. The nurse should research the drug literature before selecting option (d).**

THE PATIENT WITH AN INTESTINAL OBSTRUCTION

Mrs. W, 56 years old, is hospitalized with the diagnosis of small bowel obstruction. She has an N/G tube to low continuous suction draining dark brown drainage and an IV of D_5/0.45 NS with 30 mEq KCl infusing at 100 cc/hr. Her skin is warm and dry and her mucous membranes are dry. Her abdomen is distended with hyperactive bowel sounds in the right upper and lower quadrants. The nursing assistant reports that Mrs. W. just vomited 100 cc dark brown secretions.

Instructions: Prioritize the following **nursing interventions** as you would do them to initially take care of Mrs. W. Write a number in the box to identify the order of your interventions (#1 = first intervention, #2 = second intervention, etc.) and state a **rationale** for each intervention.

INTERVENTIONS	PRIORITY #	RATIONALE
◆ Provide thorough mouth care	☐	
◆ Assess abdomen, measure abdominal girth	☐	
◆ Assess N/G tube and suction	☐	
◆ Take the vital signs	☐	
◆ Ensure Mrs. W is in semi-Fowler's position	☐	

KEY POINTS TO CONSIDER:

After 48 hours Mrs. W's abdomen is less distended and the current assessment findings include:

1. Hgb 9.2 g, Hct 29%, K^+ 3.1 mEq , Na^+ 145 mEq
2. T. 98.8° F - P. 92, irregular - R. 20 - B/P 152/94
3. N/G tube draining dark brown drainage (250 cc in the last 8 hours)
4. Pain on a 1-10 scale = 4
5. No stool or passing of flatus, urine output last 24 hr 700 cc

✓✓✓ **Interactive activity:** With a partner, **do the following: (1) based on the current assessment, select** the **one nursing diagnosis** that is of priority at this time, **(2) provide a rationale** for your selection, and **(3) list three nursing interventions** that meet the needs of Mrs. W.

All of the following nursing diagnoses may apply to Mrs. W:

Risk for infection, Pain, Anxiety, Ineffective airway clearance, Imbalanced nutrition: less than body requirements, Deficient knowledge, Deficient fluid volume, Risk for impaired skin integrity, Fear, Disturbed sleep pattern.

Nursing Diagnosis	Rationale	Nursing Interventions
		1. 2. 3.

✓✓✓ The next day, Mrs. W's assessment included the following: N/G output 500 cc and urine output 100 cc dark amber during the night shift. Faint bowel sounds, capillary refill >5 sec. Weak, lethargic, and disoriented. Mucous membranes dry. Orthostatic B/P 148/90 (lying) 124/84 (standing).

Instructions: Based on the situation, identify and write the **priority problem** in the box below. Then, starting with the small box labeled **#1 prioritize** the **nursing interventions** for this situation and identify your follow-up action plan for Mrs. W.

NURSING INTERVENTIONS

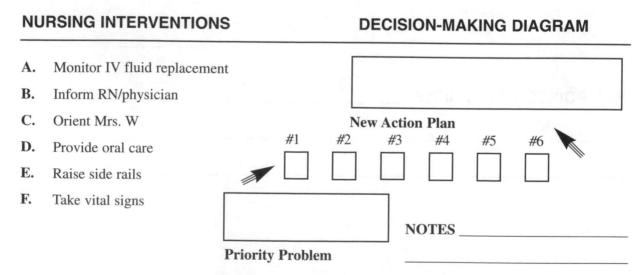

A. Monitor IV fluid replacement

B. Inform RN/physician

C. Orient Mrs. W

D. Provide oral care

E. Raise side rails

F. Take vital signs

DECISION-MAKING DIAGRAM

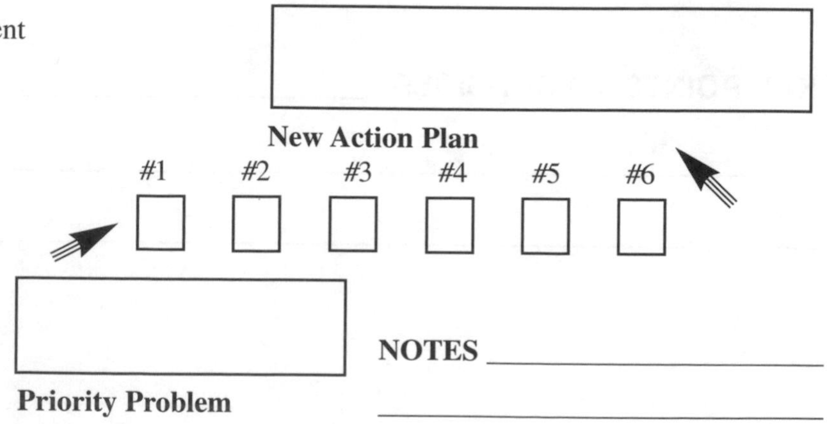

New Action Plan

#1 #2 #3 #4 #5 #6

Priority Problem

NOTES ____________

Applying Critical Thinking Skills to Test Questions

INSTRUCTIONS: Circle the one best answer for each test question. Write your rationale for selecting the answer. To enhance your learning and test-taking skill, discuss your answer and rationale with a partner. The answer and the rationale can be found on the back of this page.

1. The nurse is taking care of a client who has a nasogastric tube to continuous low suction. The nursing assistant reports that the client has vomited 100 cc of light yellow-greenish fluid. It is most important for the nurse to initially
   a. check the medication record for an anti-emetic.
   b. check the nasogastric tube placement.
   c. add the emesis to the total output for the shift.
   d. ask the client if the desire to vomit has stopped.

   Rationale: ____

2. The nurse is caring for a client who was admitted with an upper GI bleed. The client has an N/G tube to continuous low suction and has an order for Mylanta 30 cc via N/G tube q4h. The nurse administers 30 cc of Mylanta at 0900. A priority follow-up nursing intervention is to
   a. maintain the tube to low continuous suction.
   b. document medication administration.
   c. ensure nasogastric tube placement.
   d. clamp the N/G tube for 30 minutes.

   Rationale: ____

3. The client is receiving continuous full-strength formula tube feeding through a nasogastric feeding tube at 75 cc/hr and there are 100 cc left in the feeding bag. The nurse is preparing to administer the 0900 routine medications through the feeding tube. Which technique is best in administering the 0900 medications?
   a. Crush the medications, dissolve in water, and put in the feeding bag.
   b. Crush the medications, dissolve in water, and give using a 50-cc syringe.
   c. Crush the medications, dissolve in water, and check tube placement.
   d. Crush the medications, dissolve in water, and check residual before giving.

   Rationale: ____

Applying Critical Thinking Skills to Test Questions

HELPFUL HINTS: Read all test questions carefully. Identify key words in the question that will guide you in answering the question. In these test questions the **key words** to consider are **"most important," "priority,"** and **"best."** Compare your rationale with the one found for each question.

1. The nurse is taking care of a client who has a nasogastric tube to continuous low suction. The nursing assistant reports that the client has vomited 100 cc of light yellow-greenish fluid. It is most important for the nurse to initially
   a. check the medication record for an anti-emetic.
   (b.) check the nasogastric tube placement.
   c. add the emesis to the total output for the shift.
   d. ask the client if the desire to vomit has stopped.

   Rationale: **(B) is the answer. Vomiting should not be experienced with the use of an N/G tube. Tube placement should be assessed. Option (a) is not the initial intervention and options (c) and (d) are not the most important interventions.**

2. The nurse is caring for a client who was admitted with an upper GI bleed. The client has an N/G tube to continuous low suction and has an order for Mylanta 30 cc via N/G tube q4h. The nurse administers 30 cc of Mylanta at 0900. A priority follow-up nursing intervention is to
   a. maintain the tube to low continuous suction.
   b. document medication administration.
   c. ensure nasogastric tube placement.
   (d.) clamp the N/G tube for 30 minutes.

   Rationale: **(D) is the answer. It is important to clamp the tube for 30 minutes to allow for drug absorption. Option (a) is an on-going nursing action, option (b) should be done after drug administration, and option (c) should have been done before drug administration.**

3. The client is receiving continuous full-strength formula tube feeding through a nasogastric feeding tube at 75 cc/hr and there are 100 cc left in the feeding bag. The nurse is preparing to administer the 0900 routine medications through the feeding tube. Which technique is best in administering the 0900 medications?
   a. Crush the medications, dissolve in water, and put in the feeding bag.
   b. Crush the medications, dissolve in water, and give using a 50-cc syringe.
   (c.) Crush the medications, dissolve in water, and check tube placement.
   d. Crush the medications, dissolve in water, and check residual before giving.

   Rationale: **(C) is the answer. Tube placement should be checked before administration of medication or formula feeding. Options (a), (b), and (d) do not describe the best technique.**

THE PATIENT WITH A COLOSTOMY

Mrs. P, 42 years old, had surgery today for colon cancer. She was transferred to her room 2 hours ago. In the taped evening shift report you learn that she has a sigmoid colostomy with a colostomy bag in place, a clean dry surgical dressing, an N/G tube to low continuous wall suction draining dark brown drainage, a right central line with TPN infusing at 83 cc/hr, and an IV of D_5/NS with a PCA (morphine sulfate) set to deliver 1 mg/6 min per patient demand.

Instructions: Prioritize the following **nursing interventions** as you, the nurse, would do them to initially take care of Mrs. P. Write a number in the box to identify the order of your interventions (#1 = first intervention, #2 = second intervention, etc.) and state a **rationale** for each intervention.

INTERVENTIONS	PRIORITY #	RATIONALE
◆ Assess surgical dressing and stoma	☐	
◆ Take the vital signs	☐	
◆ Assess pain level	☐	
◆ Check N/G tube and drainage	☐	
◆ Check IV site, TPN and PCA setting	☐	

KEY POINTS TO CONSIDER:

The **first post-op day** assessment was significant for the following signs and symptoms:

1. Bowel sounds absent
2. Mrs. P moans when she turns in bed
3. Weak, ineffective cough
4. Stoma swollen and reddened

✓✓✓ **Interactive activity:** With a partner, **do the following: (1) select** the **one nursing diagnosis** that is of priority at this time, **(2) provide a rationale** for your selection, and **(3) list three nursing interventions** that assist to meet the needs of the patient:

All of the following nursing diagnoses may apply to Mrs. P:

Risk for infection, Risk for impaired skin integrity, Pain, Anxiety, Ineffective airway clearance, Fatigue, Impaired physical mobility, Imbalanced nutrition: less than body requirements, Disturbed body image, Risk for deficient fluid volume, Fear.

Nursing Diagnosis	Rationale	Nursing Interventions
		1. 2. 3.

✓✓✓ On the morning of the **third post-op day**, the N/G tube was removed per the physician's order and Mrs. P was started on a clear liquid diet. In the afternoon the assessment findings included:

Stoma edematous and pale, abdomen distended, c/o of pain.

Instructions: Based on the **third post-op day** assessment, identify and write the **priority problem** in the box below. Then, starting with the small box labeled **#1, prioritize** the **nursing interventions** listed and **identify** your action plan for the follow-up care of Mrs. P.

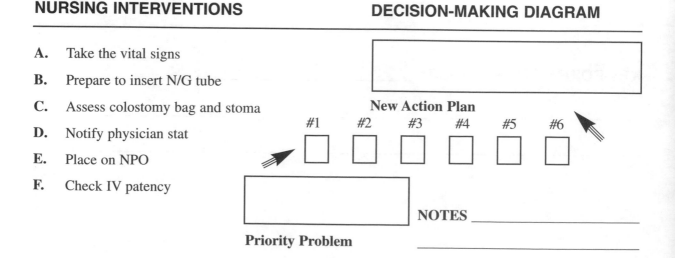

NURSING INTERVENTIONS

A. Take the vital signs

B. Prepare to insert N/G tube

C. Assess colostomy bag and stoma

D. Notify physician stat

E. Place on NPO

F. Check IV patency

DECISION-MAKING DIAGRAM

New Action Plan

#1 #2 #3 #4 #5 #6

Priority Problem

NOTES ____________

____

Applying Critical Thinking Skills to Test Questions

INSTRUCTIONS: Circle the one best answer for each test question. Write your rationale for selecting the answer. To enhance your learning and test-taking skill, discuss your answer and rationale with a partner. The answer and the rationale can be found on the back of this page.

1. The patient care rand of a client indicates that a double-barrel colostomy was performed 2 days ago. Which assessment finding is of most concern?
   a. Right-sided colostomy bag with small amount fecal drainage, left-sided colostomy bag with serosanguineous mucous drainage.
   b. Right-sided colostomy bag with serosanguineous mucous drainage. Stoma dark red. Left-sided colostomy bag with minimal drainage.
   c. Abdomen soft, tender to touch, stomas red and edematous.
   d. Bowel sounds hypoactive on right side; absent on left side.

   Rationale: ____

   ____

   ____

   ____

   ____

2. The nurse is assigned to a client who was had an ileostomy 3 days ago and now has developed rales in the upper lung fields. The client is receiving intravenous fluid set at 75 cc/hr. Which of the following interventions is most important for the nurse to ask the nursing assistant to perform?
   a. Take vital signs q4h.
   b. Monitor intake and output q8h.
   c. Push 500 cc of fluid for the shift.
   d. Assist the client to turn in bed q4h.

   Rationale: ____

   ____

   ____

   ____

   ____

3. The client is 72 years old and is admitted with a respiratory tract infection. The client is on erythromycin 400 mg q6h po. The client has a sigmoid colostomy. Which of the following assessment findings would be most indicative of a potential complication?
   a. Admission WBC of 11,500.
   b. Six liquid stools during the shift.
   c. T. 100.8° F during morning assessment.
   d. Urinary output of 260 cc for the last 4 hours.

   Rationale: ____

   ____

   ____

   ____

   ____

Applying Critical Thinking Skills to Test Questions

HELPFUL HINTS: Read all test questions carefully. Identify key words in the question that will guide you in answering the question. In these test questions the **key words** to consider are **"most concern," "most important,"** and **"most indicative."** Compare your rationale with the one found for each question.

1. The patient care rand of a client indicates that a double-barrel colostomy was performed 2 days ago. Which assessment finding is of most concern?
   a. Right-sided colostomy bag with small amount fecal drainage, left-sided colostomy bag with serosanguineous mucous drainage
   (b.) Right-sided colostomy bag with serosanguineous mucous drainage. Stoma dark red. Left-sided colostomy bag with minimal drainage
   c. Abdomen soft, tender to touch, stomas red and edematous
   d. Bowel sounds hypoactive on right side; absent on left side

   Rationale: **(B) is the answer. The dark red color of the stoma is an indication of possible impaired perfusion of the stoma. Options (a, (c), and (d) are normal assessment findings consistent with the situation.**

2. The nurse is assigned to a client who was had an ileostomy 3 days ago and now has developed rales in the upper lung fields. The client is receiving intravenous fluid set at 75 cc/hr. Which of the following interventions is most important for the nurse to ask the nursing assistant to perform?
   a. Take vital signs q4h.
   b. Monitor intake and output q8h.
   (c.) Push 500 cc of fluid for the shift.
   d. Assist the client to turn in bed q4h.

   Rationale: **(C) is the answer. A new ileostomy will initially drain up to 2 L/day. Replacing fluid to prevent dehydration is important. Options (a), (b), and (d) are good interventions, but the client needs hydration because of the fluid loss.**

3. The client is 72 years old and is admitted with a respiratory tract infection. The client is on erythromycin 400 mg q6h po. The client has a sigmoid colostomy. Which of the following assessment findings would be most indicative of a potential complication?
   a. Admission WBC of 11,500
   (b.) Six liquid stools during the shift
   c. T. 100.8° F during morning assessment.
   d. Urinary output of 260 cc for the last 4 hours.

   Rationale: **(B) is the answer. Erythromycin can cause diarrhea. With a sigmoid colostomy the client should have near-to-normal stools. Options (a) and (c) are symptoms associated with an infection, for which the client was admitted. Option (d) is WNL.**

THE PATIENT WITH COLON CANCER

Mr. S, 65 years old, has colon cancer. He is admitted for a colon resection. His current medical history is significant for complaints of changes in bowel habits/constipation, passing of bloody stools, abdominal pain, and weight loss. His past medical condition includes a history of coronary artery disease and hypertension. In addition to antihypertensive medication, he takes aspirin 81 mg po qd. In preparation for surgery, his current orders include NPO, insert an N/G tube, and a saline lock. His 6:00 AM vital signs are T. 98° F - P. 78 - R. 20 - B/P 162/90. He is to receive his pre-op medication at 12:00 PM today. The nurse gets out of report at 8:00 AM.

Instructions: Prioritize the five **nursing interventions** as you, the nurse, would do them to initially take care of Mr. S. Write a number in the box to identify the order of your interventions (#1 = first intervention, #2 = second intervention, etc.) and state a **rationale** for each intervention.

INTERVENTIONS	PRIORITY #	RATIONALE
◆ Perform a body systems assessment	☐	
◆ Take the vital signs	☐	
◆ Insert saline lock	☐	
◆ Insert N/G tube	☐	
◆ Check surgical consent	☐	

KEY POINTS TO CONSIDER: ______________________

A colon resection is done on Mr. S. The **first post-op day** assessment includes:

1. Lactated Ringer's infusing at 100 cc/hr and PCA with morphine sulfate
2. Elastic stockings on; intermittent compression device ordered for 24 hours
3. N/G tube to low continuous suction draining brown-greenish fluid
4. Wants to stay in a low Fowler's position
5. Short and shallow respirations

✓✓✓ **Interactive activity:** With a partner, **do the following: (1)** based on the **first post-op day assessment, select** the **one nursing diagnosis** that is a priority at this time, **(2) provide a rationale** for your selection, and **(3) list three nursing interventions** that meet the needs of Mr. S.

All of the following Nursing Diagnoses may apply to Mr. S:

Risk for infection, Pain, Anxiety, Ineffective airway clearance, Imbalanced nutrition: less than body requirements, Deficient knowledge, Risk for deficient fluid volume, Risk for impaired skin integrity, Risk for ineffective tissue perfusion, Fear.

Nursing Diagnosis	Rationale	Nursing Interventions
		1. 2. 3.

✓✓✓ On the **fourth postoperative day** you assess the following signs and symptoms on Mr. S:

c/o tenderness in the right calf with a positive Homan's sign, 2+ right ankle/calf edema, right calf is warmer to touch than the left calf.

Instructions: Based on the **fourth postoperative day** assessment, identify and write the **priority problem** in the box below. Then, starting with the small box labeled **#1**, **prioritize** the **nursing interventions** listed and **identify** your action plan for the follow-up care of Mr. S.

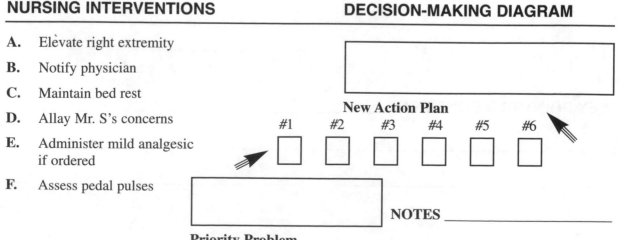

NURSING INTERVENTIONS

A. Elevate right extremity

B. Notify physician

C. Maintain bed rest

D. Allay Mr. S's concerns

E. Administer mild analgesic if ordered

F. Assess pedal pulses

DECISION-MAKING DIAGRAM

New Action Plan

#1 #2 #3 #4 #5 #6

Priority Problem

NOTES ______________

____

Applying Critical Thinking Skills to Test Questions

INSTRUCTIONS: Circle the one best answer for each test question. Write your rationale for selecting the answer. To enhance your learning and test-taking skill, discuss your answer and rationale with a partner. The answer and the rationale can be found on the back of this page.

1. The nurse is caring for a client who had a ileostomy 5 days ago. The ileostomy is draining large amounts of green-brownish liquid stool. On discharge, the client asks the nurse if the stool consistency will eventually become more solid. Which response by the nurse is best?
   a. "The stool will become solid as the ileostomy heals."
   b. "Eating certain foods can help make the stool more solid."
   c. "It takes about 1 year to see exactly what the stool consistency will be."
   d. "The stool will change to a mushy consistency after several months."

   Rationale: ____
   ____
   ____
   ____
   ____

2. The nurse is providing discharge instructions to a client who is going home after having an ileostomy for colon cancer. A priority discharge instruction is to instruct the client to
   a. irrigate the ileostomy weekly.
   b. drink eight glasses of water daily.
   c. monitor the daily output from the ileostomy.
   d. use a mild laxative if there is no ileostomy drainage for 24 hours.

   Rationale: ____
   ____
   ____
   ____
   ____

3. The nurse is assisting a client to irrigate his colostomy. After instilling the water, the client has no output. What should the nurse do next?
   a. Encourage the client to ambulate.
   b. Irrigate the colostomy again within 30 minutes.
   c. Digitally stimulate the colostomy opening.
   d. Notify the physician.

   Rationale: ____
   ____
   ____
   ____
   ____

Applying Critical Thinking Skills to Test Questions

HELPFUL HINTS: Read all test questions carefully. Identify key words in the question that will guide you in answering the question. In these test questions the **key words** to consider are **"best," "priority,"** and **"next."** Compare your rationale with the one in the test question.

1. The nurse is caring for a client who had a ileostomy 5 days ago. The ileostomy is draining large amounts of green-brownish liquid stool. On discharge, the client asks the nurse if the stool consistency will eventually become more solid. Which response by the nurse is best?
   a. "The stool will become solid as the ileostomy heals."
   b. "Eating certain foods can help make the stool more solid."
   c. "It takes about 1 year to see exactly what the stool consistency will be."
   (d.) "The stool will change to a mushy consistency after several months."

   Rationale: **(D) is the answer. Fecal drainage from an ileostomy is mostly liquid and changes to a mushy consistency in 3 to 6 months. Options (a), (b), and (c) do not provide the client with the correct information.**

2. The nurse is providing discharge instructions to a client who is going home after having an ileostomy for colon cancer. A priority discharge instruction is to instruct the client to
   a. irrigate the ileostomy weekly.
   (b.) drink eight glasses of water daily.
   c. monitor the daily output from the ileostomy.
   d. use a mild laxative if there is no ileostomy drainage for 24 hours.

   Rationale: **(B) is the answer. Daily fecal drainage from a new ileostomy can range from 1000 to 2000 ml. The client is at risk for dehydration along with fluid and electrolyte imbalance. Options (a) and (d) are interventions that do not apply to the care of an ileostomy. Option (c) is good but does not help the client prevent a complication.**

3. The nurse is assisting a client to irrigate his colostomy. After instilling the water, the client has no output. What should the nurse do next?
   (a.) Encourage the client to ambulate.
   b. Irrigate the colostomy again within 30 minutes.
   c. Digitally stimulate the colostomy opening.
   d. Notify the physician.

   Rationale: **(A) is the answer. Ambulation can stimulate peristalsis and the flow of fecal drainage. Option (b) would instill more fluid and may cause trauma and excessive loss of fluid and electrolytes. Option (c) is not appropriate and option (d) is not necessary since it may take some time for the drainage to begin.**

THE PATIENT WITH TPN

You are assigned to care for Mrs. F. In report you learn that her diarrhea is decreasing and her current VS are T. 98.8° F - P. 76 - R. 18 - B/P 130/84. She has complained of pain in her right leg.

VS q4h I & O (✓) Weigh qd BRP with assist prn Admit date: 3/16 Name: F, J. M. Age: 55	Right central line inserted 3/16 TPN @ 83 cc/hr per pump Lipids 10% (M-W-F) BS Fingersticks q6h (6-12-6-12) Dx: Dehydration/Diarrhea Hx of Crohn's-acute exacerbation, Atrial fibrillation	Diet: NPO Routine med: Vit. K 10 mg SC qMon Reg. Ins. 2 U if BS = 180 – 200 mg Call MD if BS >200 mg

Instructions: Prioritize the five **nursing interventions** as you would do them to take care of Mrs. F. Write a number in the box to identify the order of your interventions (#1 = first intervention, #2 = second intervention, etc.) and state a **rationale** for each intervention.

INTERVENTIONS	PRIORITY #	RATIONALE
◆ Perform a body systems physical assessment	☐	
◆ Assess Homan's sign	☐	
◆ Assess central line for patency and central line dressing	☐	
◆ Get 0600 blood sugar results	☐	
◆ Assess right arm and neck for distention	☐	

KEY POINTS TO CONSIDER: ______________________

Mrs. F was taken to x-ray 1 hour ago. On her return to the unit, the IV pump is beeping and you are informed that the machine has been beeping for a long time. You assess the following:

1. TPN not infusing
2. Skin warm, diaphoretic, c/o nervousness and rapid heartbeat
3. VS: T. 98° F - P. 118 - R. 26 - B/P 136/80

✓✓✓ **Interactive activity:** With a partner, **do the following: (1) select** the **one nursing diagnosis** that is of priority at this time, **(2) provide a rationale** for your selection, and **(3) list the nursing interventions** that assist to meet the needs of the patient:

All of the following nursing diagnoses may apply to Mrs. F:

Anxiety, Risk for infection, Risk for activity intolerance, Risk for excess fluid volume, Impaired tissue integrity, Ineffective tissue perfusion, Imbalanced nutrition: Less than body requirements, Risk for injury: hypoglycemia, Deficient knowledge.

Nursing Diagnosis	Rationale	Nursing Interventions
		1. **2.** **3.**

✓✓✓ **Three hours later**, Mrs. F's family calls the nursing station to say that Mrs. F is having difficulty breathing. You go into Mrs. F's room and assess the following:

c/o chest pain, R. 36 - P. 110, coughing, dyspnea, anxiousness

Instructions: Based on the **3 hours later** situation, identify and write the **priority problem** in the box below. Then, starting with the small box labeled **#1 prioritize** the **nursing interventions** for this situation and **identify** your follow-up action plan for Mrs. F.

NURSING INTERVENTIONS

A. Stay with Mrs. F

B. Raise HOB

C. Take P - R - B/P

D. Monitor O_2 saturation level

E. Notify RN/MD

F. Administer oxygen

DECISION-MAKING DIAGRAM

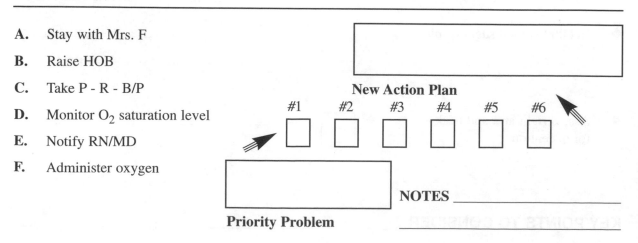

New Action Plan

#1 #2 #3 #4 #5 #6

Priority Problem

NOTES ____________________

____

THE PATIENT WITH CIRRHOSIS OF THE LIVER

Mr. U, 46 years old, was admitted with the diagnosis of Laënnec's cirrhosis. In the evening report you learn that he is jaundiced, has ascites, and is experiencing increasing SOB. His VS at 12:00 PM were T. 99° F - P. 94 - R. 34 - B/P 140/90. The vital signs are consistent with previous recordings. You get out of report at 4:30 PM. The nursing care kardex includes the following orders:

VS q4h I & O (✓) Neuro cks q4h	Saline lock (✓)	Diet: ↑ CHO, 30 g Prot., 2 g Na^+
CBC, serum ammonia } today AST, ALT, PT }	Bed rest with BRP	Routine med: Amphogel 30 cc po qid Furosemide 40 mg IV QD Aldactone 50 mg po bid
Procedure: Abd. Paracentesis at 5:00 PM today	Weigh daily Measure abd girth daily	

Instructions: Prioritize the five **nursing interventions** as you would do them to take care of Mr. U. Write a number in the box to identify the order of your interventions (#1 = first intervention, #2 = second intervention, etc.) and state a **rationale** for each intervention.

INTERVENTIONS	PRIORITY #	RATIONALE
◆ Ensure consent form is signed	☐	
◆ Take the vital signs	☐	
◆ Perform a body systems physical assessment	☐	
◆ Ensure abdominal paracentesis equipment is on the unit	☐	
◆ Have Mr. U void	☐	

KEY POINTS TO CONSIDER: ______

The physician performs the abdominal paracentesis on Mr. U and removes 2.5 L of fluid. VS during the procedure were P. 90 - R. 32 - B/P 136/86. Post-procedure you assess:

1. VS: P. 94 - R. 24 - B/P 136/86
2. Dressing at the abdominal puncture site is clean
3. Mr. U is lying in a semi-Fowler's position
4. He is alert and oriented, although slow to respond

✓✓✓ **Interactive activity:** With a partner, **do the following: (1) select** the **one nursing diagnosis** that is of priority at this time, **(2) provide a rationale** for your selection, and **(3) list the nursing interventions** that assist to meet the needs of the patient.

All of the following nursing diagnoses may apply to Mr. U:

Risk for injury: Falls, Risk for infection, Impaired skin integrity, Risk for impaired physical mobility, Pain, Imbalanced nutrition: Less than body requirements, Risk for disturbed thought processes, Risk for activity intolerance, Impaired tissue integrity, Excess fluid volume, Risk for deficient fluid volume, Ineffective breathing pattern, Disturbed body image, Disturbed sleep pattern, Fatigue, Altered comfort.

Nursing Diagnosis	Rationale	Nursing Interventions
		1. 2. 3. 4.

✓✓✓ The **laboratory results** for today are:

PT 40 sec.	Serum ammonia 70 μg/dl	Hgb 10.6 g/dl	Hct 30%
WBC 3500/mm^3	Platelets 100,000/mm^3	AST 100 U/L	ALT 500 U/L

Instructions: Based on the **laboratory results**, identify and write the **priority problem** in the box below. Then, starting with the small box labeled **#1, prioritize** the **nursing interventions** for this situation and **identify** your follow-up action plan for Mr. U.

NURSING INTERVENTIONS

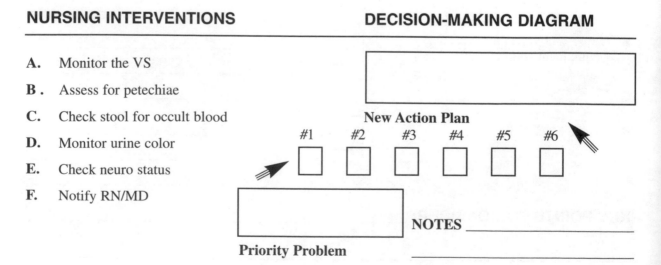

A. Monitor the VS

B. Assess for petechiae

C. Check stool for occult blood

D. Monitor urine color

E. Check neuro status

F. Notify RN/MD

DECISION-MAKING DIAGRAM

New Action Plan

#1 #2 #3 #4 #5 #6

Priority Problem

NOTES ______________

____

Applying Critical Thinking Skills to Test Questions

INSTRUCTIONS: Circle the one best answer for each test question. Write your rationale for selecting the answer. To enhance your learning and test-taking skill, discuss your answer and rationale with a partner. The answer and the rationale can be found on the back of this page.

1. The physicians order phytonadione (Vitamin K) 10 mg IM for an adult client with liver cirrhosis and ascites. Available is a vial of phytonadione 10 mg/ml. The nurse is planning to administer this dose in the deltoid. Which of the following is most appropriate for the administration of the ordered amount to the client?
   a. 1-cc syringe with 25 g ⅝″ needle
   b. 1-cc syringe with 23 g ½″ needle
   c. 3-cc syringe with 23 g 1″ needle
   d. 3-cc syringe with 22 g 1½″ needle

   Rationale: ____

2. The nurse admits a client with cirrhosis of the liver and severe ascites. The client is oriented, jaundiced, and complains of itching. Respirations are 28, short and shallow. Urine is dark amber. Which action is most important for the nurse to consider?
   a. Sit client in high-Fowler's position.
   b. Encourage client to drink more fluids.
   c. Limit client activity.
   d. Assess skin integrity qd.

   Rationale: ____

3. The client is admitted with cirrhosis of the liver and ascites. The physician orders the administration of an IV infusion of salt-poor albumin. Which of the following is the expected outcome after the administration of the salt-poor albumin?
   a. Decreased complaints of pruritis
   b. Decreased serum ammonia levels
   c. Increased secretion of sodium
   d. Increased urinary output

   Rationale: ____

Applying Critical Thinking Skills to Test Questions

HELPFUL HINTS: Read all test questions carefully. Identify key words in the question that will guide you in answering the question. In these test questions the **key words** to consider are **"most appropriate," "most important,"** and **"expected outcome."** Compare your rationale with the one in the test question.

1. The physicians order phytonadione (Vitamin K) 10 mg IM for an adult client with liver cirrhosis and ascites. Available is a vial of phytonadione 10 mg/ml. The nurse is planning to administer this dose in the deltoid. Which of the following is most appropriate for the administration of the ordered amount to the client?
   a. 1-cc syringe with 25 g ⅝″ needle
   b. 1-cc syringe with 23 g ½″ needle
   (c.) 3-cc syringe with 23 g 1″ needle
   d. 3-cc syringe with 22 g 1½″ needle

   Rationale: **(C) is the answer. It is most appropriate to use a smaller IM needle gauge since clients with liver cirrhosis are at a high risk for bleeding. The deltoid is a smaller muscle than the gluteus, so a 1-cc needle is the best choice. Options (a), (b), and (d) are not the best choice for this client.**

2. The nurse admits a client with cirrhosis of the liver and severe ascites. The client is oriented, jaundiced, and complains of itching. Respirations are 28, short and shallow. Urine is dark amber. Which action is most important for the nurse to consider?
   a. Sit client in high-Fowler's position.
   b. Encourage client to drink more fluids.
   (c.) Limit client activity.
   d. Assess skin integrity qd.

   Rationale: **(C) is the answer. Activity increases the metabolic needs of the body thereby increasing the workload of the liver. Option (a) is not the most appropriate position for a client with severe ascites since it compromises respiration. Options (b) and (d) are not the most important interventions.**

3. The client is admitted with cirrhosis of the liver and ascites. The physician orders the administration of an IV infusion of salt-poor albumin. Which of the following is the expected outcome after the administration of the salt-poor albumin?
   a. Decreased complaints of pruritis
   b. Decreased serum ammonia levels
   c. Increased secretion of sodium
   (d.) Increased urinary output

   Rationale: **(D) is the answer. Salt-poor albumin increases plasma colloid osmotic pressure thereby increasing diuresis. Options (a), (b), and (c) are not expected outcomes for this ordered intervention.**

THE PATIENT WITH HEPATIC ENCEPHALOPATHY

Mr. U, 47 years old, is admitted with the diagnosis of hepatic encephalopathy related to his advanced cirrhosis of the liver. The night report indicates that he was awake most of the night and very restless most of the shift. The nursing care kardex has the following orders:

VS q4h I & O (✓) Neuro cks q4h	D_5W at 100 cc/hr #20 g RFA - inserted today	Diet: ↑ CHO, 50 g Prot., 4 g Na^+
Serum ammonia, K^+ today	Bed rest with BRP	Routine med: Neomycin 1 g po q6h Lactulose 30 cc bid
Code Status: No code	Weigh daily	

As you enter his room you notice that Mr. U is sleeping.

Instructions: Prioritize the five **nursing interventions** as you would do them to take care of Mr. U. Write a number in the box to identify the order of your interventions (#1 = first intervention, #2 = second intervention, etc.) and state a **rationale** for each intervention.

INTERVENTIONS	PRIORITY #	RATIONALE
◆ Take the vital signs	☐	______
◆ Assess the LOC and orientation	☐	______
◆ Check current serum ammonia and K^+ levels	☐	______
◆ Perform a body systems physical assessment	☐	______
◆ Assist Mr. U with his ADLs	☐	______

KEY POINTS TO CONSIDER: ______

Mr. U has refused his morning dose of lactulose and you further assess:

1. He refused the lactulose the previous day
2. No BM for 2 days
3. Irritable, speech slurred
4. Responds slowly to verbal communication

✓✓✓ **Interactive activity:** With a partner, **do the following: (1) select** the **one nursing diagnosis** that is of priority at this time, **(2) provide a rationale** for your selection, and **(3) list the nursing interventions** that assist to meet the needs of the patient.

All of the following nursing diagnoses may apply to Mr. U:

Risk for injury: falls, Risk for infection, Impaired skin integrity, Self-care deficit: bathing/hygiene, Risk for impaired physical mobility, Risk for constipation, Imbalanced nutrition: less than body requirements, Activity intolerance, Impaired tissue integrity, Excess fluid volume, Ineffective breathing pattern, Fatigue, Disturbed thought processes, Disturbed sleep pattern, Altered comfort.

Nursing Diagnosis	Rationale	Nursing Interventions
		1. 2. 3. 4.

✓✓✓ You return from lunch at 1 PM and are informed of the following:
Mr. U is becoming increasingly confused and lethargic. He did not eat lunch.

Instructions: Based on the 1 PM information, identify and write the **priority problem** in the box below. Then, starting with the small box labeled **#1 prioritize** the **nursing interventions** for this situation and **identify** your follow-up action plan for Mr. U.

NURSING INTERVENTIONS

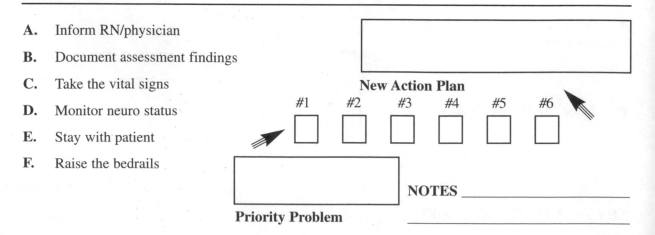

A. Inform RN/physician

B. Document assessment findings

C. Take the vital signs

D. Monitor neuro status

E. Stay with patient

F. Raise the bedrails

DECISION-MAKING DIAGRAM

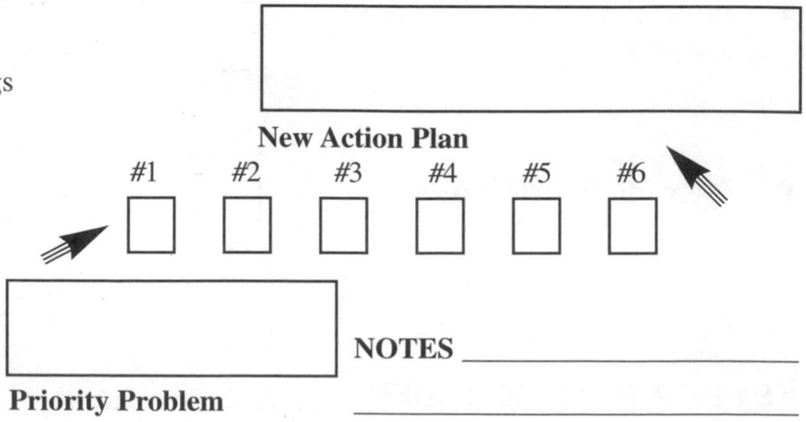

New Action Plan

#1 #2 #3 #4 #5 #6

Priority Problem

NOTES ______________________

____

Applying Critical Thinking Skills to Test Questions

INSTRUCTIONS: Circle the one best answer for each test question. Write your rationale for selecting the answer. To enhance your learning and test-taking skill, discuss your answer and rationale with a partner. The answer and the rationale can be found on the back of this page.

1. The client is diagnosed with hepatic encephalopathy and is receiving lactulose 30 ml po bid. To effectively monitor the therapeutic effects of the drug therapy, the nurse would primarily assess for a(n):
   a. decrease in abdominal girth.
   b. increase in bowel movements.
   c. increase in serum albumin levels.
   d. decrease in serum ammonia levels.

   Rationale: ____

2. The nurse administers spironolactone 100 mg po to a client with portal hypertension. Which of the following is most important for the nurse to monitor during the administration of this drug?
   a. Serum potassium levels
   b. Intake and output
   c. Specific gravity of urine
   d. Abdominal girth

   Rationale: ____

3. The nurse is caring for a client admitted with portal hypertension and ascites. Which assessment finding is most indicative of a serious complication?
   a. Caput medusae noted on abdomen
   b. Complaints of fatigue and weakness
   c. Hematemesis after breakfast
   d. 2 lb weight loss from previous day

   Rationale: ____

Applying Critical Thinking Skills to Test Questions

HELPFUL HINTS: Read all test questions carefully. Identify key words in the question that will guide you in answering the question. In these test questions the **key words** to consider are **"primarily," "most important,"** and **"most indicative."** Compare your rationale with the one in the test question.

1. The client is diagnosed with hepatic encephalopathy and is receiving lactulose 30 ml po bid. To effectively monitor the therapeutic effects of the drug therapy, the nurse would primarily assess for a(n):
   a. decrease in abdominal girth.
   b. increase in bowel movements.
   c. increase in serum albumin levels.
   (d.) decrease in serum ammonia levels.

   Rationale: **(D) is the answer. The expected therapeutic effect for this client is to decrease serum ammonia levels by trapping ammonium ions in the intestine and excreting them in the stool. Options (a) and (c) do not provide the nurse with the therapeutic drug effects, and option (b) is not as specific a measure of effectiveness as the serum ammonia level.**

2. The nurse administers spironolactone 100 mg po to a client with portal hypertension. Which of the following is most important for the nurse to monitor during the administration of this drug?
   (a.) Serum potassium levels
   b. Intake and output
   c. Specific gravity of urine
   d. Abdominal girth

   Rationale: **(A) is the answer. Serum potassium levels should be monitored when a client is on spironolactone, a potassium-sparing diuretic. Options (b), (c), and (d) are not the most important interventions.**

3. The nurse is caring for a client admitted with portal hypertension and ascites. Which assessment finding is most indicative of a serious complication?
   a. Caput medusae noted on abdomen
   b. Complaints of fatigue and weakness
   (c.) Hematemesis after breakfast
   d. 2 lb weight loss from previous day

   Rationale: **(C) is the answer. Clients with portal hypertension may also have esophageal varices. The client should be monitored for further signs of bleeding. Option (a) is a expected finding consistent with ascites. Option (b) needs further assessment, and option (d) is not most indicative of a serious complication.**

THE PATIENT WITH DIABETES MELLITUS

The nurse is assigned to a 56-year-old Hispanic female, Mrs. G, admitted with the diagnosis of end-stage renal disease. She has a 30-year history of type 1 DM. She is scheduled to have hemodialysis this AM. The night nurse indicates that she has a 2-cm dry, ulcerated circular area on the lateral outer aspect of her right great toe and an AV fistula in the right forearm. She has an order for NPH Insulin 15 U SC qAM and blood sugar fingerstick qid. It is 0730 when the nurse gets out of report and breakfast arrives on the unit at 0800.

Instructions: Prioritize the five **nursing interventions** as you would do them to initially take care of Mrs. G. Write a number in the box to identify the order of your interventions (#1 = first intervention, #2 = second intervention, etc.) and state a **rationale** for each intervention.

INTERVENTIONS	PRIORITY #	RATIONALE
◆ Check chart for blood sugar fingerstick results	☐	
◆ Assess AV fistula	☐	
◆ Administer NPH 15 U SC	☐	
◆ Get patient ready for breakfast	☐	
◆ Perform a body systems physical assessment	☐	

KEY POINTS TO CONSIDER:

Mrs. G is still waiting for her dialysis treatment. At 1000 the physician leaves the following orders:

Sliding scale - for fingerstick blood sugar:

225 - 250 give	10 U Reg Ins.
200 - 224 give	5 U Reg Ins.
150 - 199 give	2 U Reg Ins.
< 150	no insulin

You do a fingerstick at 1130. The results are 236. You will give ___________ Regular Insulin.

✓✓✓ **Interactive activity:** With a partner, **do the following: (1) select** the **one nursing diagnosis** that is a priority at this time, **(2) provide a rationale** for your selection, and **(3) list the nursing interventions** that assist you to meet the needs of the patient.

All of the following nursing diagnoses may apply to Mrs. G:

Risk for infection, Risk for impaired skin integrity, Impaired physical mobility, Altered patterns of elimination, Ineffective sexuality patterns, Disturbed sensory perception, Fatigue, Excess fluid volume, Deficient fluid volume, Imbalanced nutrition: less than body requirements

Nursing Diagnosis	Rationale	Nursing Interventions
		1. 2. 3. 4.

✓✓✓ As you take her 1300 VS you note the following signs and symptoms:
Irritability, skin warm, moist, VS: T. 36.8° C - P. 100 - R. 18 - B/P 150/84. She is c/o dizziness and "feeling funny."

Instructions: Based on the situation above, identify and write the **priority problem** in the box below. Then, starting with the small box labeled **#1 prioritize** the **nursing interventions** for this situation and **identify** your plan for follow-up care for Mrs. G.

NURSING INTERVENTIONS

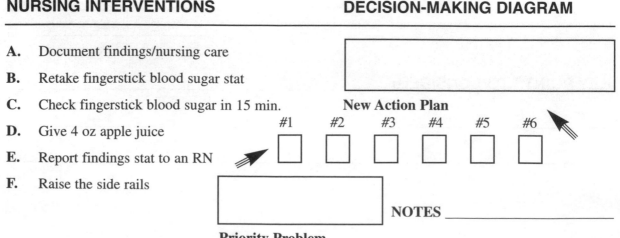

A. Document findings/nursing care

B. Retake fingerstick blood sugar stat

C. Check fingerstick blood sugar in 15 min.

D. Give 4 oz apple juice

E. Report findings stat to an RN

F. Raise the side rails

DECISION-MAKING DIAGRAM

New Action Plan

#1 #2 #3 #4 #5 #6

Priority Problem

NOTES ______________

Applying Critical Thinking Skills to Test Questions

INSTRUCTIONS: Circle the one best answer for each test question. Write your rationale for selecting the answer. To enhance your learning and test-taking skill, discuss your answer and rationale with a partner. The answer and the rationale can be found on the back of this page.

1. The nurse is providing discharge instructions to a newly diagnosed client with type 1 diabetes mellitus who will take 5 U Regular insulin and 10 U NPH insulin qAM. The client informs the nurse that he runs 2 miles every morning. In teaching the client about insulin absorption and exercise, it is important for the nurse to teach the client to
   a. inject the morning dose of insulin into the abdomen.
   b. hold the morning dose of regular insulin until after the exercise.
   c. hold the morning dose of NPH insulin until after the exercise.
   d. inject the morning dose of insulin into the lower extremity.

   Rationale: ____
   ____
   ____
   ____
   ____

2. The nurse notes the following medications on a client's medication record: Lente insulin 13 U SC q.AM at 0730 and Humalog Lispro 5 U SC at the start of breakfast. The breakfast arrives at 0830 on the unit. In assessing the medication record, which action by the nurse is most appropriate?
   a. Question the Humalog Lispro insulin order.
   b. Question the Lente insulin order.
   c. Give both insulins at 0730 in one syringe.
   d. Give the insulins as ordered.

   Rationale: ____
   ____
   ____
   ____
   ____

3. The nurse is preparing to draw up NPH 12 U using a low-dose insulin syringe. Which technique indicates the most appropriate procedure before giving the insulin? The nurse takes the medication record and the syringe with the 12 U of insulin and
   a. checks the drawn-up dose with another nurse.
   b. with the syringe in the vial, checks the drawn-up dose with another nurse.
   c. takes the vial of insulin to check the drawn-up dose with another nurse.
   d. double checks by charting the dose of insulin before injecting the insulin.

   Rationale: ____
   ____
   ____
   ____
   ____

Applying Critical Thinking Skills to Test Questions

HELPFUL HINTS: Read all test questions carefully. Identify key words in the question that will guide you in answering the question. In these test questions the **key words** to consider are **"absorption and exercise"** and **"most appropriate."** Compare your rationale with the one in the test question.

1. The nurse is providing discharge instructions to a newly diagnosed client with type 1 diabetes mellitus who will take 5 U Regular insulin and 10 U NPH insulin qAM. The client informs the nurse that he runs 2 miles every morning. In teaching the client about insulin absorption and exercise, it is important for the nurse to teach the client to
   - (a.) inject the morning dose of insulin into the abdomen.
   - b. hold the morning dose of regular insulin until after the exercise.
   - c. hold the morning dose of NPH insulin until after the exercise.
   - d. inject the morning dose of insulin into the lower extremity.

   Rationale: **(A) is the answer. The abdomen is a better injection site since the absorption rate of insulin is faster when injected into an extremity that is exercised. Options (b), (c), and (d) do not correlate the effects of diabetes, insulin therapy, and exercise.**

2. The nurse notes the following medications on a client's medication record: Lente insulin 13 U SC q.AM at 0730 and Humalog Lispro 5 U SC at the start of breakfast. The breakfast arrives at 0830 on the unit. In assessing the medication record, which action by the nurse is most appropriate?
   - a. Question the Humalog Lispro insulin order.
   - b. Question the Lente insulin order.
   - c. Give both insulins at 0730 in one syringe.
   - (d.) Give the insulins as ordered.

   Rationale: **(D) is the answer. It is most appropriate to consider that Humalog Lispro is a rapid-acting insulin with an onset of 10 to 15 minutes and should be administered at the start of the meal. Options (a), (b), and (c) do not address the onset of action of the rapid-acting insulin.**

3. The nurse is preparing to draw up NPH 12 U using a low-dose insulin syringe. Which technique indicates the most appropriate procedure before giving the insulin? The nurse takes the medication record and the syringe with the 12 U of insulin and
   - a. checks the drawn-up dose with another nurse.
   - (b.) with the syringe in the vial, checks the drawn-up dose with another nurse.
   - c. takes the vial of insulin to check the drawn-up dose with another nurse.
   - d. double checks by charting the dose of insulin before injecting the insulin.

   Rationale: **(B) is the answer. To prevent a medication error, it is recommended that the syringe remain in the insulin vial when checking the type and dose of insulin with another nurse. Options (a), (c), and (d) are not the most appropriate and recommended procedure.**

THE PATIENT UNDERGOING HEMODIALYSIS

Ms. A, 52 years old, has ESRD and has just been started on dialysis. She has an AV fistula in the right forearm and is scheduled for dialysis at 0800 today. The night nurse reports that the fistula has a good thrill and bruit. Ms. A's B/P is 160/102. You leave the report room at 0730 after noting the following orders from the nursing care kardex:

VS q8h I & O (✓) Weigh daily H & H, Serum Ferritin (✓) Serum Iron Saturation (✓)	IV: Saline lock - left hand Routine medications: Vasotec 10 mg po qd 0800 Folic acid 1 mg po qd 0800 FeSo 4 325 po tid c̄ meals Epogen 30,000 U SC M-W-F	Diet: 70 g Protein, 2 g Na^+, 2 g K^+ Fluid restriction 1000 cc/day

Instructions: Prioritize the five **nursing interventions** as you would do them to take care of Ms. A. Write a number in the box to identify the order of your interventions (#1 = first intervention, #2 = second intervention, etc.) and state a **rationale** for each intervention.

INTERVENTIONS	PRIORITY #	RATIONALE
◆ Take the VS (B/P on the left arm)	☐	
◆ Perform body systems physical assessment	☐	
◆ Weigh patient/ensure patient has been weighed	☐	
◆ Assess AV fistula for thrill and bruit	☐	
◆ Hold folic acid and Vasotec	☐	

KEY POINTS TO CONSIDER:

Ordered laboratory studies were drawn before dialysis. The results of the morning laboratory tests are:

1. Hgb 9.5 g/dl, Hct 28%
2. Ferritin 60 ng/L
3. Serum iron saturation 18%
4. K^+ 5.0 mEq

✓✓✓ **Interactive activity:** With a partner, **do the following: (1) select** the **one nursing diagnosis** that is of priority at this time, **(2) provide a rationale** for your selection, and **(3) list the nursing interventions** that assist to meet the needs of the patient.

All of the following nursing diagnoses may apply to Ms. A:

Risk for injury, Deficient knowledge, Fear, Anxiety, Risk for infection, Impaired tissue integrity, Risk for disturbed sensory perception, Constipation, Excess fluid volume, Deficient fluid volume, Disturbed body image, Risk for impaired physical mobility, Ineffective tissue perfusion, Imbalanced nutrition: less than body requirements, Fatigue.

Nursing Diagnosis	Rationale	Nursing Interventions
		1. **2.** **3.** **4.**

✓✓✓ **After the dialysis treatment**, Ms. A is restless and you assess:

c/o headache, pruritis, nausea, change in LOC, twitching, confusion

Instructions: Based on **after the dialysis treatment data**, identify and write the **priority problem** in the box below. Then, starting with the small box labeled **#1 prioritize** the **nursing interventions** for this situation and **identify** your follow-up action plan for Ms. A.

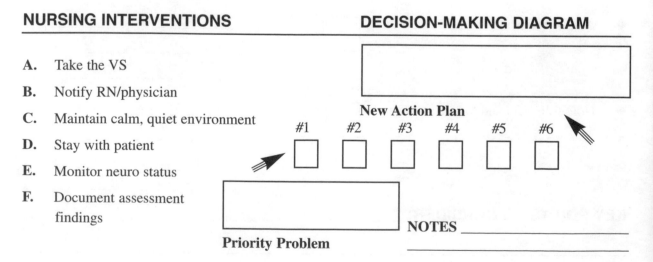

NURSING INTERVENTIONS

A. Take the VS

B. Notify RN/physician

C. Maintain calm, quiet environment

D. Stay with patient

E. Monitor neuro status

F. Document assessment findings

DECISION-MAKING DIAGRAM

New Action Plan

#1 #2 #3 #4 #5 #6

Priority Problem

NOTES ______________

Applying Critical Thinking Skills to Test Questions

INSTRUCTIONS: Circle the one best answer for each test question. Write your rationale for selecting the answer. To enhance your learning and test-taking skill, discuss your answer and rationale with a partner. The answer and the rationale can be found on the back of this page.

1. The client with end-stage renal disease related to type 1 diabetes mellitus has completed hemodialysis 1 hour ago. Which nursing intervention is of priority in assisting the alert adult client to transfer from the bed to the chair post-dialysis?
   a. Check the blood glucose level.
   b. Monitor for dizziness on standing.
   c. Wrap the AV fistula with gauze.
   d. Do not move the arm with the AV fistula.

   Rationale: ____

2. The nurse administers Epoetin10,000 U SC to the client with end-stage renal disease twice weekly. The most effective method of evaluating the therapeutic effect of Epoetin is for the nurse to assess for
   a. a decrease in skin pallor.
   b. an increase in client activity.
   c. an increase in the hematocrit level.
   d. a decrease in complaints of weakness and fatigue.

   Rationale: ____

3. The nurse is caring for a client scheduled for hemodialysis this morning. In preparing the client for the dialysis treatment, it is most important for the nurse to
   a. allow the client to rest until after the dialysis treatment.
   b. ensure that all morning care is completed before dialysis.
   c. make the client NPO until after the dialysis treatment.
   d. withhold the morning dose of any antihypertensive drugs.

   Rationale: ____

Applying Critical Thinking Skills to Test Questions

HELPFUL HINTS: Read all test questions carefully. Identify key words in the question that will guide you in answering the question. In these test questions the **key words** to consider are **"priority," "most effective,"** and **"most important."** Compare your rationale with the one in the test question.

1. The client with end-stage renal disease related to type 1 diabetes mellitus has completed hemodialysis 1 hour ago. Which nursing intervention is of priority in assisting the alert adult client to transfer from the bed to the chair post-dialysis?
   a. Check the blood glucose level.
   (b.) Monitor for dizziness on standing.
   c. Wrap the AV fistula with gauze.
   d. Do not move the arm with the AV fistula.

   Rationale: **(B) is the answer. Hypotension is a complication post-dialysis related to the rapid removal of fluid. The nurse should monitor for orthostatic changes. Options (a) and (c) are important but not of priority post-dialysis. Option (d) is an intervention that can apply to a new fistula.**

2. The nurse administers Epoetin10,000 U SC to the client with end-stage renal disease twice weekly. The most effective method of evaluating the therapeutic effect of Epoetin is for the nurse to assess for
   a. a decrease in skin pallor.
   b. an increase in client activity.
   (c.) an increase in the hematocrit level.
   d. a decrease in complaints of weakness and fatigue.

   Rationale: **(C) is the answer. Epoetin stimulates the production of RBCs. The hematocrit (hct) is an indirect measurement of the total number and volume of RBCs. Options (a), (b), and (d) may be manifested as a result of the rise in the number of red blood cells.**

3. The nurse is caring for a client scheduled for hemodialysis this morning. In preparing the client for the dialysis treatment, it is most important for the nurse to
   a. allow the client to rest until after the dialysis treatment.
   b. ensure that all morning care is completed before dialysis.
   c. make the client NPO until after the dialysis treatment.
   (d.) withhold the morning dose of any antihypertensive drugs.

   Rationale: **(D) is the answer. Hypotension is a complication of dialysis. Antihypertensive drugs taken before dialysis can cause severe hypotension. Options (a) and (b) are not the most important in preparing the client, and option (c) is not necessary in preparing the client for hemodialysis.**

THE PATIENT WITH PERIPHERAL ARTERIAL DISEASE

Mr. L, 70 years old, is sent to the hospital after visiting his physician with c/o increasing painful muscle cramps after ambulating. He lives alone, and his medical history is significant for hypertension.

The nursing care kardex has the following admit orders:

VS q4h I & O (✓) Pedal pulse check q4h Bed rest with BRP CBC Mr. L Age: 70	Insert Saline lock Drsg chgs: Clean ulcerated area on left foot with NS - apply dry sterile 4 × 4s Dx. Peripheral Arterial Disease	Diet: Mech Soft Routine med: Trental 400 mg po tid Dipyridamole 50 mg po tid

You are assigned to begin his admission. You note that he is alert but hard of hearing. He has a bandage around his left foot. He tells you he uses this to keep his shoe from rubbing his foot.

Instructions: Prioritize the five **nursing interventions** as you would do them to take care of Mr. L. Write a number in the box to identify the order of your interventions (#1 = first intervention, #2 = second intervention, etc.) and state a **rationale** for each intervention.

INTERVENTIONS	PRIORITY #	RATIONALE
◆ Take the vital signs	☐	______
◆ Assess bilateral pedal pulses	☐	______
◆ Orient to hospital room	☐	______
◆ Perform a body systems assessment	☐	______
◆ Apply sterile dressing to left foot	☐	______

KEY POINTS TO CONSIDER: ______

You assist Mr. L to the bathroom; on his return to bed you note the following:

1. Bilateral lower extremities—reddish blue in color
2. Bilateral pedal pulses weak (1+), capillary refill > 3 sec.
3. Lower extremities cool to touch
4. Gait slow, needs assistance

✓✓✓ **Interactive activity:** With a partner, **do the following: (1) select** the **one nursing diagnosis** that is of priority at this time, **(2) provide a rationale** for your selection, and **(3) list the nursing interventions** that assist to meet the needs of the patient.

All of the following nursing diagnoses may apply to Mr. L:

Risk for injury: fall, Deficient knowledge, Risk for infection, Impaired skin integrity, Self-care deficit, Risk for impaired physical mobility, Ineffective peripheral tissue perfusion, Activity intolerance, Impaired tissue integrity, Pain.

Nursing Diagnosis	Rationale	Nursing Interventions
		1. 2. 3. 4.

✓✓✓ You **remove the bandage** from the left foot and you note:

A circular ulcerated area with two toes blackened and shriveled

Instructions: Based on **removal of the bandage** information, identify and write the **priority problem** in the box below. Then, starting with the small box labeled **#1 prioritize** the **nursing interventions** for this situation and **identify** your follow-up action plan for Mr. L.

NURSING INTERVENTIONS

A. Notify RN/physician

B. Measure ulcerated area

C. Put sterile gloves on

D. Cleanse area with NS

E. Apply sterile dressing

F. Document assessment findings

DECISION-MAKING DIAGRAM

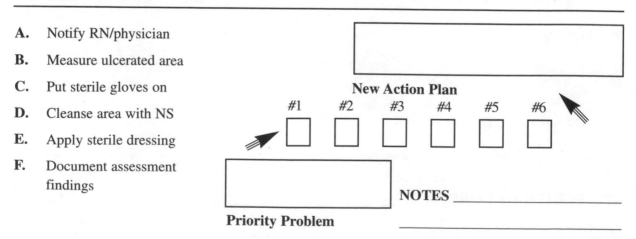

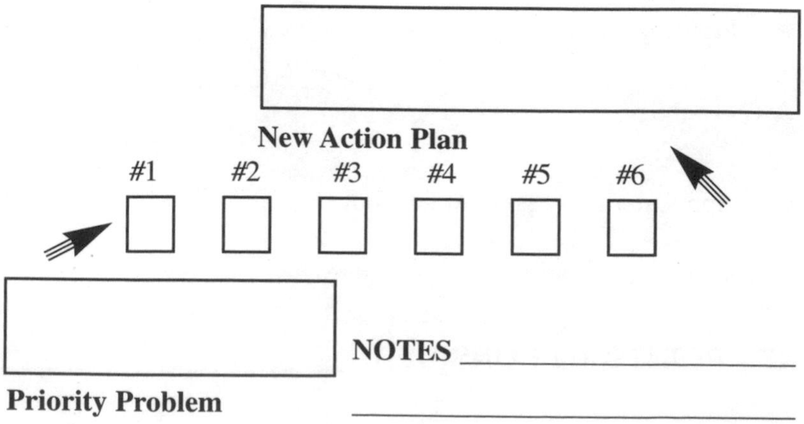

New Action Plan

#1 #2 #3 #4 #5 #6

Priority Problem

NOTES ____________

THE PATIENT WITH CHEST PAIN

Mrs. T, 56 years old, was admitted after experiencing chest pain. She has coronary artery disease and smokes 1 pack of cigarettes a day. Her father died of heart disease and she has a brother with hypertension. Her VS are T. 98° F - P. 90 - R. 26 - B/P 164/100. Mrs. T has been taking verapamil, Procardia, and Tenormin. Mrs. T will continue with her usual cardiac and blood pressure medications and is also started on baby aspirin, Colace, and Lovastatin. Nitroglycerin tablets 0.4 mg SL are ordered prn chest pain and Mylanta 30 cc q2h prn. She has BRP with assistance, a saline lock, and oxygen at 2-3 L/NC to keep O_2 sat >96%. The night nurse reports that Mrs.T is upset about not being able to smoke. Mrs. T is requesting to use the commode as you start your shift.

Instructions: Prioritize the five **nursing interventions** as you would do them to initially take care of Mrs. T. Write a number in the box to identify the order of your interventions (#1 = first intervention, #2 = second intervention, etc.) and state a **rationale** for each intervention.

INTERVENTIONS	PRIORITY #	RATIONALE
◆ Take the vital signs	☐	________
◆ Assist to commode	☐	________
◆ Perform a body systems assessment	☐	________
◆ Check O_2 saturation level	☐	________
◆ Talk with Mrs. T	☐	________

KEY POINTS TO CONSIDER: ________________________________

____

____

After breakfast Mrs. T continues to be upset. She states that she is constipated and above all wants to smoke. She is getting increasingly upset. You observe the following:

1. Abdomen round, bowel sounds present in all four quadrants
2. Breakfast intake 30%
3. LBM 2 days ago
4. O_2 saturation level 93%

✓✓✓ **Interactive activity:** With a partner, **do the following: (1) select** the **one nursing diagnosis** that is of priority at this time, **(2) provide a rationale** for your selection, and **(3) list the nursing interventions** that assist to meet the needs of the patient.

All of the following nursing diagnoses may apply to Mrs. T:

Pain, Deficient knowledge, Anxiety, Risk for noncompliance, Risk for decreased cardiac output, Activity intolerance, Ineffective tissue perfusion: cardiopulmonary, Risk for impaired skin integrity, Constipation, Ineffective health maintenance.

Nursing Diagnosis	Rationale	Nursing Interventions
		1. 2. 3. 4.

✓✓✓ At **10:00 AM** the nursing assistant reports that Mrs. T is experiencing chest pain. You assess and note that she has cool, clammy skin, c/o tightness in the chest with pain radiating to the left arm, B/P 154/98, P. 100, R. 30. O_2 is at 2 L/nasal cannula, O_2 sat 88%.

Instructions: Based on the data at **10:00 AM**, identify and write the **priority problem** in the box below. Then, starting with the small box labeled **#1 prioritize** the **nursing interventions** for this situation and **identify** your follow-up action plan for Mrs. T.

NURSING INTERVENTIONS

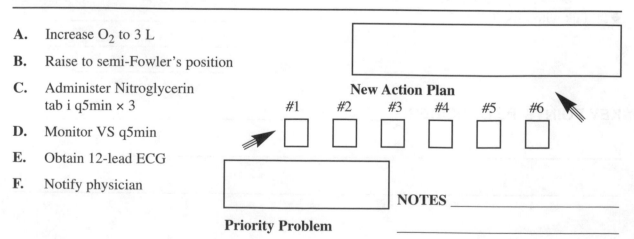

A. Increase O_2 to 3 L

B. Raise to semi-Fowler's position

C. Administer Nitroglycerin tab i q5min × 3

D. Monitor VS q5min

E. Obtain 12-lead ECG

F. Notify physician

DECISION-MAKING DIAGRAM

New Action Plan

#1 #2 #3 #4 #5 #6

Priority Problem

NOTES ____________

THE PATIENT WITH CHF

You are assigned to Mr. T who was transferred to your unit earlier today. In report you learn that he has CHF, 3+ pitting edema of the lower extremities, increasing SOB and has been demonstrating Cheyne-Stokes respirations, periods of confusion, and c/o blurred vision.
Vital signs are T. 97.6° F - P. 62 - R. 22 - B/P 180/102. He has received his 0900 meds. Current orders include:

VS q4h I & O (✓) Up in chair QID O_2 @ 3L/NP Serum K+, PT, PTT, ABG (✓) Chest x-ray (✓) ECG (✓) Name: T. Age: 72	IV D5W @ 50 cc/hr IV site: LFA #20 g LBM: 2 days ago Foley (✓) Code Status: Full code Dx: CHF	Diet: Soft (NAS) Routine medications: Digoxin 0.25 mg IV qAM 0900 Furosemide 40 mg po bid 0900-1700 Docusate sodium tab i po qAM 0900 Minipress 10 mg po bid 0900-1700

Instructions: Prioritize the five **nursing interventions** as you would do them to take care of Mr. T. Write a number in the box to identify the order of your interventions (#1 = first intervention, #2 = second intervention, etc.) and state a **rationale** for each intervention.

INTERVENTIONS	PRIORITY #	RATIONALE
◆ Assess respiratory rate	☐	
◆ Obtain urinary output data	☐	
◆ Assess rate/rhythm and quality of pulse	☐	
◆ Assess c/o visual disturbances	☐	
◆ Check current lab data	☐	

KEY POINTS TO CONSIDER: __________

Mr. T wants to wash up, but he says that he does not have the energy like he used to and that he gets tired very easily. You assess the following:

1. Skin cool, dusky in color
2. Lower extremities with 2+ pitting edema
3. Lung sounds with crackles on inspiration; R. 24 - regular pattern
4. Alert and oriented at this time

✓✓✓ **Interactive activity:** With a partner, **do the following: (1) select** the **one nursing diagnosis** that is of priority at this time, **(2) provide a rationale** for your selection, and **(3) list the nursing interventions** that assist you to meet the needs of the patient.

All of the following nursing diagnoses may apply to Mr. T:

Anxiety, Risk for infection, Activity intolerance, Excess fluid volume, Impaired tissue integrity, Risk for ineffective tissue perfusion: cerebral, Imbalanced nutrition: less than body requirements, Risk for injury, Deficient knowledge, Impaired gas exchange, Fatigue

Nursing Diagnosis	Rationale	Nursing Interventions
		1. **2.** **3.** **4.**

✓✓✓ Mr. T's family stops to visit during lunch. **At 1:00 PM**, the nursing assistant tells you that Mr. T is in distress. You walk into the room and notice Mr. T holding his chest tightly. Shortly after you assess: cyanosis, no pulse, no B/P, and no respirations.

Instructions: Based on the **1:00 PM** situation, identify and write the **priority problem** in the box below. Then, starting with the small box labeled **#1 prioritize** the **nursing interventions** for this situation and **identify** your follow-up action plan for Mr. T.

NURSING INTERVENTIONS

A. Call a code

B. Place in supine position

C. Begin CPR

D. Notify physician

E. Document findings

F. Support family

DECISION-MAKING DIAGRAM

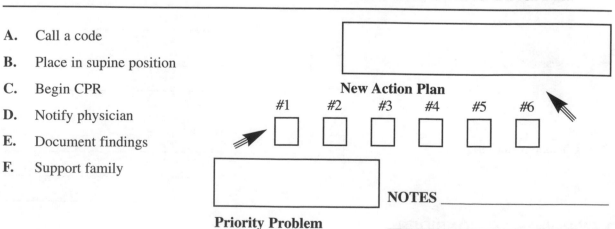

New Action Plan

#1 #2 #3 #4 #5 #6

Priority Problem

NOTES ________________

Applying Critical Thinking Skills to Test Questions

INSTRUCTIONS: Circle the one best answer for each test question. Write your rationale for selecting the answer. To enhance your learning and test-taking skill, discuss your answer and rationale with a partner. The answer and the rationale can be found on the back of this page.

1. The nurse admits a 69-year-old male client experiencing congestive heart failure. The doctor orders furosemide 60 mg IV stat, digoxin 0.25 mg po, and KCl 20 mEq p.o. now. Which assessment finding is most indicative of an ineffective response 2 hours after the administration of all the medications?
   a. Pulse 89, irregular
   b. Urine output 60 cc
   c. Pulse oximetry 94%
   d. Pitting edema in the lower extremities

   Rationale: ______________________________

2. The home health nurse visits a client with congestive heart failure. In reviewing the client's medications, the nurse notes that the client takes the following daily oral medications: digoxin 0.25 mg, furosemide 10 mg, and captopril 0.625 mg. After speaking to the client and wife, the nurse suspects digitalis toxicity. Which question helps the nurse gather more information specific to digitalis toxicity?
   a. "Do you get light-headed when you get out of bed?"
   b. "Do you need to sleep with more than one pillow?"
   c. "Do you have to get up to urinate more frequently?"
   d. "Have you had any nausea, vomiting, or diarrhea?"

   Rationale: ______________________________

3. The nurse is assigned to a client with congestive heart failure. The nurse's morning lung assessment indicates crackles and wheezes in the mid to lower lung bases, R 32, client restless. Which nursing intervention is of priority initially?
   a. Assess capillary refill
   b. Take the pulse oximetry
   c. Limit client activity
   d. Assess fluid intake

   Rationale: ______________________________

Applying Critical Thinking Skills to Test Questions

HELPFUL HINTS: Read all test questions carefully. Identify key words in the question that will guide you in answering the question. In these test questions the **key words** to consider are **"most indicative," "specific information,"** and **"priority initially."** Compare your rationale with the one in the test question.

1. The nurse admits a 69-year-old male client experiencing congestive heart failure. The doctor orders furosemide 60 mg IV stat, digoxin 0.25 mg po, and KCl 20 mEq p.o. now. Which assessment finding is most indicative of an ineffective response 2 hours after the administration of all the medications?
   a. Pulse 89, irregular
   (b.) Urine output 60 cc
   c. Pulse oximetry 94%
   d. Pitting edema in the lower extremities

   Rationale: **(B) is the answer. Although output falls within the parameters of renal function, the client received furosemide IV and diuresis is the desired effect. Options (a), (c), and (d) are expected findings in a client with CHF.**

2. The home health nurse visits a client with congestive heart failure. In reviewing the client's medications, the nurse notes that the client takes the following daily oral medications: digoxin 0.25 mg, furosemide 10 mg, and captopril 0.625 mg. After speaking to the client and wife, the nurse suspects digitalis toxicity. Which question helps the nurse gather more information specific to digitalis toxicity?
   a. "Do you get light-headed when you get out of bed?"
   b. "Do you need to sleep with more than one pillow?"
   c. "Do you have to get up to urinate more frequently?"
   (d.) "Have you had any nausea, vomiting, or diarrhea?"

   Rationale: **(D) is the answer. Although these signs and symptoms are frequently seen with all drug therapy, they are frequently early side effects of digitalis toxicity. Options (a), (b), and (c) relate to the action of the other drugs.**

3. The nurse is assigned to a client with congestive heart failure. The nurse's morning lung assessment indicates crackles and wheezes in the mid to lower lung bases, R 32, client restless. Which nursing intervention is of priority initially?
   a. Assess capillary refill
   (b.) Take the pulse oximetry
   c. Limit client activity
   d. Assess fluid intake

   Rationale: **(B) is the answer. Client assessment indicates rapid breathing and possible hypoxia. To fully assess the respiratory status of the client, it is important to take the pulse oximetry. Options (a), (c), and (d) are important, but not priority interventions.**

THE PATIENT WITH A CVA

Mr. H, 68 years old, suffered a right-sided CVA. He was admitted to the telemety unit 2 days ago and he has been on heparin therapy. The latest documentation in the nursing notes shows: Hand grips R > L, speech slurred, B/P 166/102. The orders in the nursing care kardex include:

VS q4h I & O (✓) Neuro checks q4h Up in chair today O_2 @ 2L/NP Hospital day: #3	IV: 500cc D5W/with heparin 10,000 U infuse at 1000 U/hr Foley (✓) Foley care bid ROM to Left side Serum K^+, Na^+ & CBC today PTT daily	Diet: Full liquid Swallowing precautions Routine med: Docusate sodium 5 cc po qd Nimodipine 20 mg po tid

You begin your shift and during report you learn that Mr. H had a restful night and there were no changes in his condition. You prepare to assist Mr. H with his breakfast.

Instructions: Prioritize the five **nursing interventions** as you would do them to take care of Mr. H. Write a number in the box to identify the order of your interventions (#1 = first intervention, #2 = second intervention, etc.) and state a **rationale** for each intervention.

INTERVENTIONS	PRIORITY #	RATIONALE
◆ Place in high-Fowler's position	☐	
◆ Place food on right side for patient to see	☐	
◆ Place food into unaffected side of mouth	☐	
◆ Check inside of mouth for food caught between gums and teeth (pocketing)	☐	
◆ Use thickened liquids	☐	

KEY POINTS TO CONSIDER: ______________________________

As morning care is given to Mr. H you assess the following:

1. Does not turn head if spoken to from left side
2. Left hand/arm elevated on a pillow
3. Passive ROM is performed to extremities on the left side
4. Anti-embolic stockings on
5. Lack of awareness of left side

✓✓✓ **Interactive activity:** With a partner, **do the following: (1) select** the **one nursing diagnosis** that is of priority at this time, **(2) provide a rationale** for your selection, and **(3) list the nursing interventions** that assist you to meet the needs of the patient.

All of the following nursing diagnoses may apply to Mr. H:

Risk for injury: Falls, Deficient knowledge, Fear, Anxiety, Risk for infection, Impaired tissue integrity, Disturbed sensory perception, Constipation, Impaired swallowing, Impaired verbal communication, Self-care deficit: bathing/hygiene, Impaired urinary elimination, Disturbed body image, Risk for impaired physical mobility, Ineffective tissue perfusion, Unilateral neglect, Risk for aspiration, Risk for disuse syndrome

Nursing Diagnosis	Rationale	Nursing Interventions
		1. 2. 3.

✓✓✓ **Mr. H's lab** data is called to the unit. The results are:

PTT 250 sec (control 38 sec), K^+ 3.5 mEq, Na^+ 145 mEq, Hgb 11.4 g/dl, Hct 34%, Platelets 110,000/mm^3

Instructions: Based on **Mr. H's lab** data, identify and write the **priority problem** in the box below. Then, starting with the small box labeled **#1 prioritize** the **nursing interventions** for this situation and **identify** your follow-up action plan for Mr. H.

NURSING INTERVENTIONS

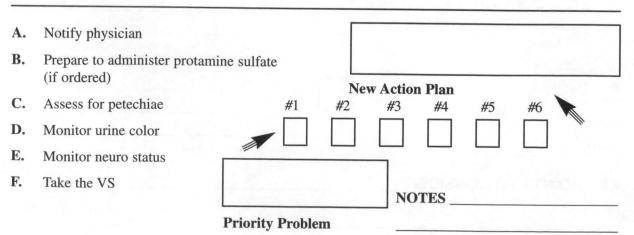

A. Notify physician
B. Prepare to administer protamine sulfate (if ordered)
C. Assess for petechiae
D. Monitor urine color
E. Monitor neuro status
F. Take the VS

DECISION-MAKING DIAGRAM

New Action Plan

#1 #2 #3 #4 #5 #6

Priority Problem

NOTES ____________

Applying Critical Thinking Skills to Test Questions

INSTRUCTIONS: Circle the one best answer for each test question. Write your rationale for selecting the answer. To enhance your learning and test-taking skill, discuss your answer and rationale with a partner. The answer and the rationale can be found on the back of this page.

1. The nurse is caring for a client who had a right-sided CVA 5 days ago and is experiencing unilateral neglect. In delegating the care of the client, which nursing intervention is of priority? The nurse instructs the nursing assistant to
   a. have the client use a communication board.
   b. place the food tray to the right side of the body.
   c. remind the client to look at the left side of the body.
   d. provide passive ROM to the left side of the body.

   Rationale: ____

2. The nurse walks into a client's room. The client is in supine position and the wife is stroking his hand. The client had a left-sided CVA 7 days ago, is on a dysphagic diet, and has an indwelling urinary catheter. Which nursing action is of priority for this client?
   a. Raise the head of the bed.
   b. Encourage the wife to talk softly to the client.
   c. Remind the client to look and touch the affected side.
   d. Assess the color and amount of output.

   Rationale: ____

3. The nurse is preparing to administer oral medications to a client who is on a dysphagic diet. Which nursing action is best in administering the medications to the client. Crush the medications and
   a. put the crushed medications in 15 cc tap water.
   b. mix the crushed medications in 4 oz of applesauce.
   c. dissolve the crushed medications in 30 cc warm water.
   d. mix the crushed medications in 30 cc thickened liquid.

   Rationale: ____

Applying Critical Thinking Skills to Test Questions

HELPFUL HINTS: Read all test questions carefully. Identify key words in the question that will guide you in answering the question. In these test questions the **key words** to consider are **"priority"** and **"best."** Compare your rationale with the one in the test question.

1. The nurse is caring for a client who had a right-sided CVA 5 days ago and is experiencing unilateral neglect. In delegating the care of the client, which nursing intervention is of priority? The nurse instructs the nursing assistant to
   a. have the client use a communication board.
   b. place the food tray to the right side of the body.
   (c.) remind the client to look at the left side of the body.
   d. provide passive ROM to the left side of the body.

   Rationale: **(C) is the answer. Clients who have a right-sided CVA experience spatial and perceptual deficits. Clients will neglect the left side of the body. Options (a), (b), and (d) do not correlate the clients need to the intervention.**

2. The nurse walks into a client's room. The client is in supine position and the wife is stroking his hand. The client had a left-sided CVA 7 days ago, is on a dysphagic diet, and has an indwelling urinary catheter. Which nursing action is of priority for this client?
   (a.) Raise the head of the bed.
   b. Encourage the wife to talk softly to the client.
   c. Remind the client to look and touch the affected side.
   d. Assess the color and amount of output.

   Rationale: **(A) is the answer. The potential for aspiration is a serious concern. Every nursing measure should be implemented to prevent this complication. Options (b), (c), and (d) are important, but they are not priorities at this time.**

3. The nurse is preparing to administer oral medications to a client who is on a dysphagic diet. Which nursing action is best in administering the medications to the client. Crush the medications and
   a. put the crushed medications in 15 cc tap water.
   b. mix the crushed medications in 4 oz of applesauce.
   c. dissolve the crushed medications in 30 cc warm water.
   (d.) mix the crushed medications in 30 cc thickened liquid.

   Rationale: **(D) is the answer. Use a small amount of thickened liquids to mix and administer the medications. Options (a) and (c) are not appropriate since water may cause the client to aspirate. Option (b) is mixing the medications in too large a quantity of apple sauce.**

THE PATIENT WITH COPD

You are assigned to Mr. Y, a 61-year-old male who has COPD. In the morning report you learn that he has been agitated during the night and is dyspneic this morning. The 0600 vital signs are T. 98.8° F - P. 102 - R. 32 - B/P 146/98. His 0700 pulse oximeter reading was 89% (room air) and he has an aminophylline drip infusing at 6 mg/hr per controller and O_2 at 2L/NC. He receives albuterol inhaler 2 puffs q4h and Atrovent inhaler 2 puffs q4h. He had a serum theophylline level drawn in the evening. You get out of report at 0730.

Instructions: Prioritize the five **nursing interventions** as you would do them to initially take care of Mr. Y. Write a number in the box to identify the order of your interventions (#1 = first intervention, #2 = second intervention, etc.) and state a **rationale** for each intervention.

INTERVENTIONS	PRIORITY #	RATIONALE
◆ Auscultate lung sounds	☐	______
◆ Assess pulse oximeter, O_2, and NC	☐	______
◆ Retake the vital signs	☐	______
◆ Check theophylline level	☐	______
◆ Place in high-Fowler's position	☐	______

KEY POINTS TO CONSIDER: ______

______

______

As you provide morning care to Mr. Y you note the following signs and symptoms:

1. Nonproductive cough; long expiratory phase during respiration
2. Increased SOB with mild exertion
3. Crackles audible throughout the bilateral lung fields
4. Anxious and restless
5. Theophylline level 14 μg/ml

✓✓✓ **Interactive activity:** With a partner, **do the following: (1) select** the **one nursing diagnosis** that is of priority at this time, **(2) provide a rationale** for your selection, and **(3) list the nursing interventions** that assist to meet the needs of the patient.

All of the following nursing diagnoses may apply to Mr. Y:

Ineffective breathing pattern, Ineffective airway clearance, Risk for injury, Risk for infection, Anxiety, Impaired gas exchange, Activity intolerance, Risk for impaired skin integrity, Imbalanced nutrition: less than body requirements, Sexual dysfunction

Nursing Diagnosis	Rationale	Nursing Interventions
		1. **2.** **3.**

✓✓✓ At **12:00 PM** the patient care assistant reports that Mr. Y is very warm and that his VS are T. 102° F - P. 98 - R. 32 - B/P 140/84. He is expectorating thick yellow-colored sputum.

Instructions: Based on the **12:00 PM** situation, identify and write the **priority problem** in the box below. Then, starting with the small box labeled **#1 prioritize** the **nursing interventions** for this situation and **identify** your follow-up action plan for Mr. Y.

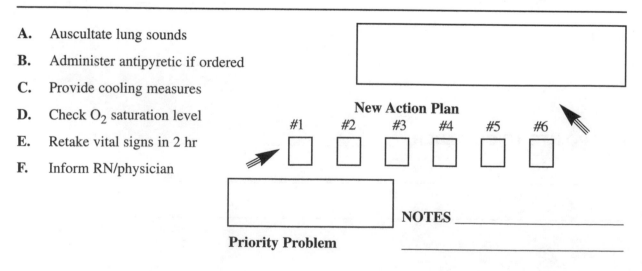

NURSING INTERVENTIONS **DECISION-MAKING DIAGRAM**

A. Auscultate lung sounds

B. Administer antipyretic if ordered

C. Provide cooling measures

D. Check O_2 saturation level

E. Retake vital signs in 2 hr

F. Inform RN/physician

New Action Plan

#1 #2 #3 #4 #5 #6

Priority Problem

NOTES ______________________

____

Applying Critical Thinking Skills to Test Questions

INSTRUCTIONS: Circle the one best answer for each test question. Write your rationale for selecting the answer. To enhance your learning and test-taking skill, discuss your answer and rationale with a partner. The answer and the rationale can be found on the back of this page.

1. The nurse is caring for a client who was admitted with an exacerbation of COPD. The client's respirations are 28 with dyspnea on exertion. The client is receiving 2 L of oxygen per nasal cannula. The morning pulse oximetry is 92%. Which nursing intervention is of priority?
   a. Monitor the client.
   b. Notify the physician.
   c. Get an order to increase the oxygen.
   d. Place in semi-Fowler's position.

   Rationale: ______________________________

2. The client has a long history of COPD and is currently experiencing an exacerbation of COPD. The following lab work is done this morning: CBC, ABGs and an electrolyte panel consisting of K^+, Na^+, Cl, CO_2, BUN, and FBS. Which lab data require immediate follow-up?
   a. PaO_2 WNL
   b. Increased RBCs
   c. Increased $PaCO_2$
   d. Hgb WNL

   Rationale: ______________________________

3. The client is admitted with an acute exacerbation of COPD. Which assessment finding is most indicative of a potential complication?
   a. R. 32, increasingly anxious and restless
   b. Using accessory muscles during respiration
   c. Pulse oximetry 92%, purse-lip breathing
   d. Expectorating copious amount of white phlegm

   Rationale: ______________________________

Applying Critical Thinking Skills to Test Questions

HELPFUL HINTS: Read all test questions carefully. Identify key words in the question that will guide you in answering the question. In these test questions the **key words** to consider are **"priority," "immediate,"** and **"most indicative."** Compare your rationale with the one in the test question.

1. The nurse is caring for a client who was admitted with an exacerbation of COPD. The client's respirations are 28 with dyspnea on exertion. The client is receiving 2 L of oxygen per nasal cannula. The morning pulse oximetry is 92%. Which nursing intervention is of priority?
   (a.) Monitor the client.
   b. Notify the physician.
   c. Get an order to increase the oxygen.
   d. Place in semi-Fowler's position.

   Rationale: **(A) is the answer. The client is manifesting signs and symptoms consistent with COPD. Clients with COPD experience some degree of hypoxia. Options (b) and (c) are not appropriate at this time. Option (d) is not the best position for a client with COPD.**

2. The client has a long history of COPD and is currently experiencing an exacerbation of COPD. The following lab work is done this morning: CBC, ABGs and an electrolyte panel consisting of K^+, Na^+, Cl, CO_2, BUN, and FBS. Which lab data require immediate follow-up?
   (a.) PaO_2 WNL
   b. Increased RBCs
   c. Increased $PaCO_2$
   d. Hgb WNL

   Rationale: **(A) is the answer. Hypoxemia provides the stimulus for the respiratory drive in client with COPD. Increased oxygen levels may depress the respiratory drive. Options (b) and (c) are expected findings. Option (d) does not require immediate follow-up.**

3. The client is admitted with an acute exacerbation of COPD. Which assessment finding is most indicative of a potential complication?
   (a.) R. 32, increasingly anxious and restless
   b. Using accessory muscles during respiration
   c. Pulse oximetry 92%, purse-lip breathing
   d. Expectorating copious amount of white phlegm

   Rationale: **(A) is the answer. Increasing anxiousness and restlessness are signs indicating hypoxemia. Options (b), (c), (d) are expected findings for a client with an exacerbation of COPD.**

THE PATIENT WITH A CHEST TUBE

Mr. G, 23 years old, has been in the hospital for 2 days after being stabbed in the chest. He has a posterior chest tube connected to a Pleu-evac system. You are assigned to his care and the nursing care kardex contains the following information:

VS q4h I & O (✓) Amb with assist prn O_2 @ 2-3L/NP/Pulse ox q4h Chest tube to low con't suction	IV: D5/0.45 NS q12h IVPB Cefazolin 1G IV q6h Chest x-ray today ABG today	Diet: Soft Routine med: Colace 100 mg po qd

7:00 AM report indicates that he had a restful night. Chest tube drainage was 15 cc. Midnight VS are T. 99° F - P. 90 - R. 22 - B/P 128/74. Pulse oximetry at 4:00 AM was 95%.

Instructions: Prioritize the five **nursing interventions** as you would do them to take care of Mr. G. Write a number in the box to identify the order of your interventions (#1 = first intervention, #2 = second intervention, etc.) and state a **rationale** for each intervention.

INTERVENTIONS	PRIORITY #	RATIONALE
◆ Check the pulse oximetry	☐	______
◆ Assess for fluctuation in the water-seal chamber and bubbling in the suction-control chamber	☐	______
◆ Check for the previous shift's fluid level marking on the tape	☐	______
◆ Assess chest tube patency and drainage	☐	______
◆ Ask Mr. G to cough and deep breathe	☐	______

KEY POINTS TO CONSIDER: ______

After breakfast, Mr. G is transported to the x-ray department via wheelchair. On his return to his room you assess the following:

1. VS: T. 99.8° F - P. 92 - R. 26 - B/P 140/90
2. c/o dyspnea, crackles auscultated, anxious
3. O_2 off, O_2 saturation level 88%

✓✓✓ **Interactive activity:** With a partner, **do the following: (1) select** the **one nursing diagnosis** that is of priority at this time, **(2) provide a rationale** for your selection, and **(3) list the nursing interventions** that assist you to meet the needs of the patient.

All of the following nursing diagnoses may apply to Mr. G:

Ineffective airway clearance, Ineffective breathing pattern, Impaired gas exchange, Risk for injury, Deficient knowledge, Fear, Anxiety, Risk for infection, Impaired tissue integrity

Nursing Diagnosis	Rationale	Nursing Interventions
		1. **2.** **3.** **4.** **5.**

✓✓✓ **One hour later**, Mr. G becomes increasingly restless and, as you take his vital signs, he pulls out the chest tube.

Instructions: Based on the **1 hour later** situation, identify and write the **priority problem** in the box below. Then, starting with the small box labeled **#1 prioritize** the **nursing interventions** for this situation and **identify** your follow-up action plan for Mr. G.

NURSING INTERVENTIONS

A. Instruct Mr. G to take a deep breath and hold

B. Cover chest tube site with petroleum jelly and 4 x 4 gauze

C. Apply gloves

D. Increase O_2 to 3L

E. Notify RN/physician

F. Pinch chest tube site together

DECISION-MAKING DIAGRAM

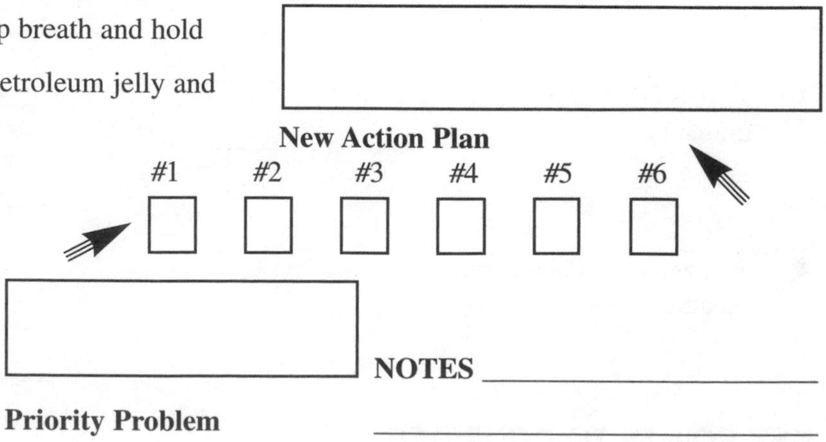

New Action Plan

#1 #2 #3 #4 #5 #6

Priority Problem

NOTES ______________________

____

Applying Critical Thinking Skills to Test Questions

INSTRUCTIONS: Circle the one best answer for each test question. Write your rationale for selecting the answer. To enhance your learning and test-taking skill, discuss your answer and rationale with a partner. The answer and the rationale can be found on the back of this page.

1. The nurse is preparing to assist with the insertion of a chest tube that will be attached to a closed-chest drainage system without suction. In monitoring the closed-chest drainage system, the nurse would expect to initially assess for
   a. fluctuation of water in the water-seal chamber during respirations.
   b. constant fluid fluctuations in the drainage-collection chamber.
   c. continuous bubbling in the suction-control chamber.
   d. occasional bubbling in the suction-control chamber.

   Rationale: ____
   ____
   ____
   ____
   ____

2. The client has a chest tube connected to a closed-chest drainage system attached to suction and is being prepared to transfer to another room on a stretcher. To safely transport the client, it is most important for the nurse to
   a. clamp the chest tube during the transport.
   b. get a portable suction before transferring the client.
   c. keep the closed-chest drainage system below the level of the chest.
   d. place the closed-chest drainage system next to the client on the stretcher.

   Rationale: ____
   ____
   ____
   ____
   ____

3. The physician is preparing to remove the client's chest tube. Just before removing the chest tube, the physician tells the client to take a deep breath and hold it. The intervention is primarily done to
   a. distract the client during the chest tube removal.
   b. minimize the negative pressure within the pleural space.
   c. decrease the degree of discomfort to the client.
   d. increase the intrathoracic pressure temporarily during removal.

   Rationale: ____
   ____
   ____
   ____
   ____

Applying Critical Thinking Skills to Test Questions

HELPFUL HINTS: Read all test questions carefully. Identify key words in the question that will guide you in answering the question. In these test questions the **key words** to consider are **"initially," "most important,"** and **"primarily."** Compare your rationale with the one in the test question.

1. The nurse is preparing to assist with the insertion of a chest tube that will be attached to a closed-chest drainage system without suction. In monitoring the closed-chest drainage system, the nurse would expect to initially assess for
   (a.) fluctuation of water in the water-seal chamber during respirations.
   b. constant fluid fluctuations in the drainage-collection chamber.
   c. continuous bubbling in the suction-control chamber.
   d. occasional bubbling in the suction-control chamber.

   Rationale: **(A) is the answer. Fluctuations of water during inspiration and expiration inthe water-seal chamber indicates normal functioning. Option (b) should not be seen in the collection chamber. Options (c) and (d) should not be seen since suction has not been applied to the suction-control chamber.**

2. The client has a chest tube connected to a closed-chest drainage system attached to suction and is being prepared to transfer to another room on a stretcher. To safely transport the client, it is most important for the nurse to
   a. clamp the chest tube during the transport.
   b. get a portable suction before transferring the client.
   (c.) keep the closed-chest drainage system below the level of the chest.
   d. place the closed-chest drainage system next to the client on the stretcher.

   Rationale: **(C) is the answer. Keeping the closed-chest drainage system below the level of the chest allows for continuous drainage and prevents any back flow pressure. Options (a) and (d) should not be done because they will increase pressure in the pleural space. Option (b) is not the most important.**

3. The physician is preparing to remove the client's chest tube. Just before removing the chest tube, the physician tells the client to take a deep breath and hold it. The intervention is primarily done to
   a. distract the client during the chest tube removal.
   b. minimize the negative pressure within the pleural space.
   c. decrease the degree of discomfort to the client.
   (d.) increase the intrathoracic pressure temporarily during removal.

   Rationale: **(D) is the answer. This is done to decrease the risk of atmospheric air entering the pleural space during removal. Options (a) and (c) are not the primary reasons for this intervention. Option (b) is not correct since negative pressure is desired within the lung.**

THE PATIENT WITH UROSEPSIS

Mr. TD, 79 years old, was admitted today to the hospital with the diagnosis of urosepsis. He has an IV of D_5/0.45 NS infusing at 100 cc/hr. Rocephin 1 g IVPB qd is ordered. He is on I & O q8h, soft diet, BRP with assistance and Tylenol tabs ii po q4h for temperature >38°C. The day shift nurse indicated his VS were T. 38° C - P. 78 - R. 22 - B/P 146/88 at 2:00 PM. The nurse also said that he was more restless this afternoon and had been trying to get out of bed and seemed somewhat disoriented. He did not receive Tylenol but an order for a vest restraint was obtained and has been applied. You have been assigned as his nurse for the evening shift.

Instructions: Prioritize the following **nursing interventions** as you, the nurse, would do them to initially take care of Mr. TD. Write a number in the box to identify the order of your interventions (#1 = first intervention, #2 = second intervention, etc.) and state a **rationale** for each intervention.

INTERVENTIONS	PRIORITY #	RATIONALE
◆ Administer Tylenol tabs ii po if necessary	☐	______
◆ Take the vital signs	☐	______
◆ Gather urinary output data	☐	______
◆ Check the vest restraint	☐	______
◆ Perform a body systems physical assessment	☐	______

KEY POINTS TO CONSIDER: ______

______

______

You perform a follow-up assessment at 7:00 PM and note the following:

1. VS: T. 38.5° C - P. 88 - R. 22 - B/P 120/76
2. Fine crackles audible on auscultation in the bilateral lower lung fields
3. He is sleepy
4. He was incontinent of a scant amount of urine

✓✓✓ **Interactive activity:** With a partner, **do the following: (1) select** the **one nursing diagnosis** that is of priority at this time, **(2) provide a rationale** for your selection, and **(3) list the nursing interventions** that assist to meet the needs of the patient.

All of the following nursing diagnoses may apply to Mr. TD:

Risk for impaired skin integrity, Impaired urinary elimination, Risk for injury, Disturbed thought processes, Hyperthermia, Deficient fluid volume, Imbalanced nutrition: less than body requirements, Ineffective breathing pattern, Fatigue

Nursing Diagnosis	Rationale	Nursing Interventions
		1. **2.** **3.** **4.** **5.**

✓✓✓ As you take his **8:00 PM** vital signs you note the following signs and symptoms:

Lethargic, skin very warm and flushed, VS: T. 39.1° C - P. 130 - R. 28 - B/P 90/54

Instructions: Based on the **8:00 PM** situation above, identify and write the **priority problem** in the box below. Then, starting with the small box labeled **#1 prioritize** the **nursing interventions** for this situation and **identify** your follow-up action plan for Mr. TD.

NURSING INTERVENTIONS

A. Check oxygen saturation level

B. Place in modified Trendelenburg position

C. Prepare to insert indwelling urinary catheter

D. Take vital signs

E. Document findings

F. Notify RN/physician

DECISION-MAKING DIAGRAM

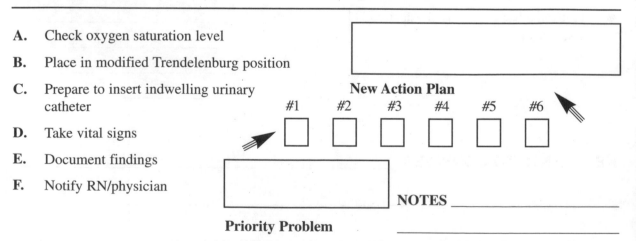

New Action Plan

#1 #2 #3 #4 #5 #6

Priority Problem

NOTES ____________________

____

THE PATIENT WITH A TURP

Mr. J, 68 years old, had a TURP this morning after having been diagnosed with benign prostatic hypertrophy. The following post-op orders have been noted:

VS q4h I & O - qs Antiembolic hose × 24 hr Sequential teds × 24 hr Up in chair this PM	IV: RL @ 100cc/hr IV site: RFA # 20g 3-way urinary catheter to gravity with continuous irrigation of NS to keep UA free of clots	Diet: Clear liquids this PM PRN Medication: B&O supp. q4h prn bladder spasms

As you enter his room you notice that his urinary drainage bag is almost full and the normal saline irrigation bag is empty.

Instructions: Prioritize the five **nursing interventions** as you would do them to take care of Mr. J. Write a number in the box to identify the order of your interventions (#1 = first intervention, #2 = second intervention, etc.) and state a **rationale** for each intervention.

INTERVENTIONS	PRIORITY #	RATIONALE
◆ Take the vital signs	☐	______
◆ Assess continuous urinary irrigation system	☐	______
◆ Empty urinary drainage bag	☐	______
◆ Perform a body systems physical assessment	☐	______
◆ Hang up new normal saline irrigation bag	☐	______

KEY POINTS TO CONSIDER: ______

On the first post-op day you assess the following on Mr. J:

1. VS: T. 99.6° F - P. 88 - R. 20 - B/P 150/88
2. Urine pinkish, no clots
3. Grimaces and says, "I didn't think it would be this tough."
4. Urinary catheter taped to thigh

✓✓✓ **Interactive activity:** With a partner, **do the following: (1) select** the **one nursing diagnosis** that is of priority at this time, **(2) provide a rationale** for your selection, and **(3) list the nursing interventions** that assist you to meet the needs of the patient.

All of the following nursing diagnoses may apply to Mr. J:

Risk for infection, Impaired tissue integrity, Excess fluid volume, Deficient knowledge, Anxiety, Risk for injury, Impaired urinary elimination, Pain, Ineffective sexuality patterns, Self-esteem, situational, low, Ineffective tissue perfusion

Nursing Diagnosis	Rationale	Nursing Interventions
		1. 2. 3.

✓✓✓ The normal saline irrigation is discontinued at 12:00 PM the first post-op day. Toward the end of the shift (**3:00 PM**), you **assess** the following on Mr. J:

c/o pain, no output since 12:00 PM, abdominal distention, and Mr. J is somewhat restless.

Instructions: Based on the **3:00 PM assessment**, identify and write the **priority problem** in the box below. Then, starting with the small box labeled **#1 prioritize** the **nursing interventions** for this situation and **identify** your follow-up action plan for Mr. J.

NURSING INTERVENTIONS

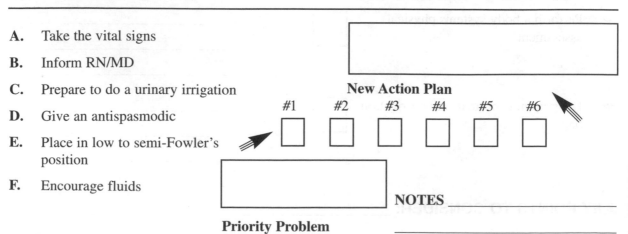

A. Take the vital signs

B. Inform RN/MD

C. Prepare to do a urinary irrigation

D. Give an antispasmodic

E. Place in low to semi-Fowler's position

F. Encourage fluids

DECISION-MAKING DIAGRAM

New Action Plan

#1 #2 #3 #4 #5 #6

Priority Problem

NOTES ________________

Applying Critical Thinking Skills to Test Questions

INSTRUCTIONS: Circle the one best answer for each test question. Write your rationale for selecting the answer. To enhance your learning and test-taking skill, discuss your answer and rationale with a partner. The answer and the rationale can be found on the back of this page.

1. The client is one day post-op transurethral resection of the prostate. He has a three-way indwelling urinary catheter with continuous bladder irrigation. During change of shift report, the nurse learns that the client's output was 1700 cc. A priority nursing intervention is for the nurse to
   a. check the client's oral and parenteral intake for the previous shift.
   b. know the amount of irrigation fluid that infused during the previous shift.
   c. assess if the client has passed any urinary clots through the catheter.
   d. ensure that the urinary output is yellow to pinkish in color.

   Rationale: ____

2. The doctor orders continuous bladder irrigation for a client who had a transurethral resection of the prostate this morning. To effectively implement this order, it is most important for the nurse to infuse the irrigation solution
   a. to maintain urine output clear to light pink in color.
   b. when the urine is red with visible clots.
   c. so that the intake equals the output.
   d. at a rate of 50 cc/hr.

   Rationale: ____

3. The client is two days post-op transurethral resection of the prostate and is complaining of an increasing urge to void. The client has a three-way urinary catheter with continuous bladder irrigation. After assessing that the catheter is patent and is draining freely, the priority nursing intervention is to
   a. reassure the client that the catheter is draining appropriately.
   b. document the client's complaints and assessment findings.
   c. give the client antispasmodic medication.
   d. notify the physician.

   Rationale: ____

Applying Critical Thinking Skills to Test Questions

HELPFUL HINTS: Read all test questions carefully. Identify key words in the question that will guide you in answering the question. In these test questions the **key words** to consider are **"priority"** and **"most important."** Compare your rationale with the one in the test question.

1. The client is one day post-op transurethral resection of the prostate. He has a three-way indwelling urinary catheter with continuous bladder irrigation. During change of shift report, the nurse learns that the client's output was 1700 cc. A priority nursing intervention is for the nurse to
   a. check the client's oral and parenteral intake for the previous shift.
   (b.) know the amount of irrigation fluid that infused during the previous shift.
   c. assess if the client has passed any urinary clots through the catheter.
   d. ensure that the urinary output is yellow to pinkish in color.

   Rationale: **(B) is the answer. It is important to know the amount of irrigation solution that infused in order to assess the actual urinary output. Options (a), (c), and (d) are good interventions, but not of priority.**

2. The doctor orders continuous bladder irrigation for a client who had a transurethral resection of the prostate this morning. To effectively implement this order, it is most important for the nurse to infuse the irrigation solution
   (a.) to maintain urine output clear to light pink in color.
   b. when the urine is red with visible clots.
   c. so that the intake equals the output.
   d. at a rate of 50 cc/hr.

   Rationale: **(A) is the answer. Continuous irrigation is given to prevent clot formation and prevent obstruction of the catheter. Options (b), (c), and (d) are not appropriate interventions.**

3. The client is two days post-op transurethral resection of the prostate and is complaining of an increasing urge to void. The client has a three-way urinary catheter with continuous bladder irrigation. After assessing that the catheter is patent and is draining freely, the priority nursing intervention is to
   a. reassure the client that the catheter is draining appropriately.
   b. document the client's complaints and assessment findings.
   (c.) give the client antispasmodic medication.
   d. notify the physician.

   Rationale: **(C) is the answer. Bladder spasms can cause the client to experience an urge to void. Options (a) and (b) do not address the client's current need. Option (d) is not appropriate at this time.**

THE PATIENT RECEIVING A BLOOD TRANSFUSION

Mr. TA, 34 years old, was admitted following a motor vehicle accident: pedestrian vs car. He sustained multiple injuries throughout his body. He will receive two units of whole blood this morning. He has NS 0.9% infusing at TKO rate through a Y-shaped blood administration set, and he has a 19g cannula in the RFA. The MD orders to infuse each unit over 3-4 hours. As you get out of the report the lab notifies you that the first unit of blood is ready.

Instructions: Prioritize the five **nursing interventions** as you would do them to take care of Mr. TA. Write a number in the box to identify the order of your interventions (#1 = first intervention, #2 = second intervention, etc.) and state a **rationale** for each intervention.

INTERVENTIONS	PRIORITY #	RATIONALE
◆ Take an initial set of vital signs	☐	
◆ Pick up the blood from the lab	☐	
◆ Assess the IV site	☐	
◆ Start the transfusion	☐	
◆ Verify MD order, patient ID, and blood compatability	☐	

KEY POINTS TO CONSIDER:

You assess the following during the start of the transfusion on Mr. TA:

1. VS: T. 97.6° F - P. 80 - R. 18 - B/P 136/78 (pre-transfusion)
2. VS: T. 98.2° F - P. 90 - R. 22 - B/P 130/70 (15 minutes after the start of the transfusion)
3. No complaints of itching
4. Transfusion rate increased to 100 cc/hr

✓✓✓ **Interactive activity:** With a partner, **do the following: (1) select** the **one nursing diagnosis** that is of priority at this time, **(2) provide a rationale** for your selection, and **(3) list the nursing interventions** that assist to meet the needs of the patient.

All of the following nursing diagnoses may apply to Mr. TA:

Risk for infection, Fatigue, Excess fluid volume, Deficient fluid volume, Deficient knowledge, Anxiety, Risk for injury, Pain

Nursing Diagnosis	Rationale	Nursing Interventions
		1. 2. 3.

✓✓✓ After 20 minutes Mr. TA's **assessment** includes:

Skin flushed, P. 120 - R. 32 - B/P 100/60, c/o chest pain and chills

Instructions: Based on the **assessment** above, identify and write the **priority problem** in the box below. Then, starting with the small box labeled **#1 prioritize** the **nursing interventions** for this situation and **identify** your follow-up action plan for Mr. TA.

NURSING INTERVENTIONS **DECISION-MAKING DIAGRAM**

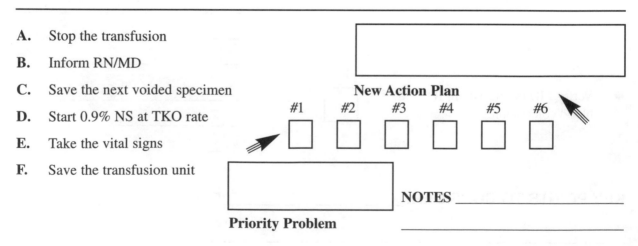

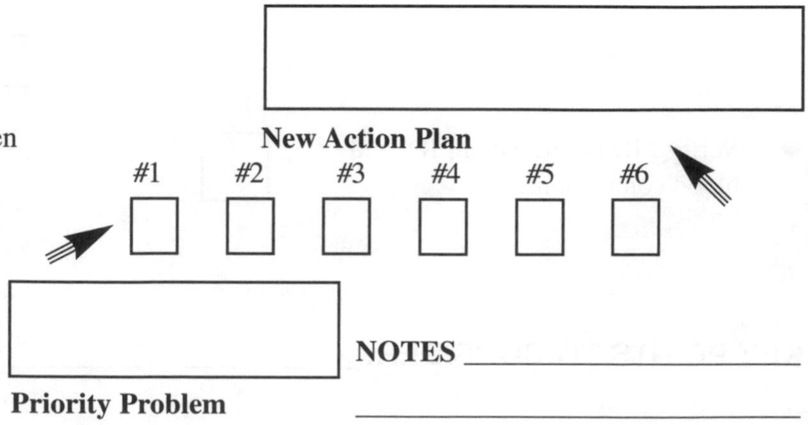

A. Stop the transfusion

B. Inform RN/MD

C. Save the next voided specimen

D. Start 0.9% NS at TKO rate

E. Take the vital signs

F. Save the transfusion unit

New Action Plan

#1 #2 #3 #4 #5 #6

Priority Problem

NOTES ____________

THE PATIENT WITH NEUTROPENIA

Mrs. K, 50 years old, was admitted 2 days ago with neutropenia. Her current WBC is 750/mm^3. During morning report you note the following from the nursing care kardex:

VS q4h I & O Neutropenic precautions (✓) Bone marrow biopsy - today CBC with diff - today Chest x-ray done	Diet: ↑ protein, ↑ calorie (no raw vegetables/fresh fruit) IV: D_5W @ 125cc/hr IV site: RFA (inserted 2 days ago)	Routine Medication: Colace 100 mg po qd 0900 PRN Medication: Tylenol 325 tabs ii q4h po prn temp >100.4° F

Instructions: Prioritize the five **nursing interventions** as you would do them to take care of Mrs. K. Write a number in the box to identify the order of your interventions (#1 = first intervention, #2 = second intervention, etc.) and state a **rationale** for each intervention.

INTERVENTIONS	PRIORITY #	RATIONALE
◆ Wash hands	☐	______
◆ Assess the IV site	☐	______
◆ Provide fresh water at bedside	☐	______
◆ Assess oral mucosa	☐	______
◆ Take the vital signs	☐	______

KEY POINTS TO CONSIDER: ______

Mrs. K is diagnosed with acute leukemia. Your follow-up assessment includes:

1. Hgb 9.8 g/dl, Hct 29%
2. WBC 900/mm^3
3. Using ordered antifungal medication as ordered
4. Platelet count 100,000/mm^3

✓✓✓ **Interactive activity:** With a partner, **do the following: (1) select** the **one nursing diagnosis** that is of priority at this time, **(2) provide a rationale** for your selection, and **(3) list the nursing interventions** that assist to meet the needs of the patient.

All of the following nursing diagnoses may apply to Mrs. K:

Risk for infection, Fatigue, Imbalanced nutrition: less than body requirements, Deficient knowledge, Anxiety, Risk for injury, Impaired oral mucous membrane, Activity intolerance, Risk for impaired skin integrity, Social isolation, Ineffective tissue perfusion

Nursing Diagnosis	Rationale	Nursing Interventions
		1. **2.** **3.** **4.**

✓✓✓ The following day, Mrs. K's **assessment findings** are significant for:

Platelet count 30,000/mm^3; bleeding time prolonged, oral petechiae, hemoptysis, tachypnea, dyspnea, and a current nosebleed.

Instructions: Based on the **assessment** above, identify and write the **priority problem** in the box below. Then, starting with the small box labeled **#1 prioritize** the **nursing interventions** for this situation and **identify** your follow-up action plan for Mrs. K.

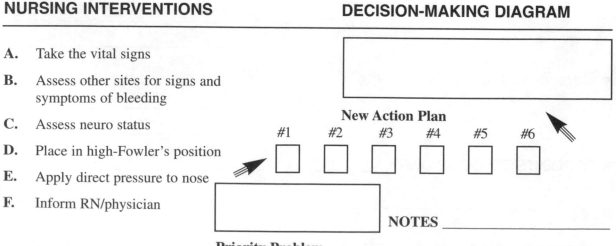

NURSING INTERVENTIONS

A. Take the vital signs

B. Assess other sites for signs and symptoms of bleeding

C. Assess neuro status

D. Place in high-Fowler's position

E. Apply direct pressure to nose

F. Inform RN/physician

DECISION-MAKING DIAGRAM

New Action Plan

#1 #2 #3 #4 #5 #6

Priority Problem

NOTES ______________

THE PATIENT WITH A HIP FRACTURE

Mrs. T, 72 years old, fell at home and was admitted to the hospital with a fracture of the right hip. She was alert and oriented on admission. After the initial work-up she was taken to surgery for an open reduction with internal fixation (ORIF) of her right hip. On her first post-op day, her right hip dressing has a small amount of dried dark red drainage. She has an IV of D_5/0.45 NS at 75 cc/hr, O_2 at 2L/NC, clear liquid diet and circulation, movement, sensation, and temperature (CMST) neurovascular checks q4h to the right leg for the first 24 hr. The following medications are ordered: Meperidine 50 mg IM q3-4h prn pain, $FeSo_4$ 325 mg po tid with meals (start when on regular diet), Colace 100 mg po qd. She is very restless and confused this morning.

Instructions: Prioritize the five interventions according to Mrs. T's current needs. Write a number in the box to identify the order of your interventions (#1 = first intervention, #2 = second intervention, etc.) and state a **rationale** for each intervention.

INTERVENTIONS	PRIORITY #	RATIONALE
◆ Assess surgical dressing	☐	
◆ Take the vital signs	☐	
◆ Assess pain level	☐	
◆ Check O_2 saturation level	☐	
◆ Check neuro status of right leg (CMST)	☐	

KEY POINTS TO CONSIDER:

During the follow-up assessment for the **first post-op day** you note the following:

1. Pedal pulse present; weak in the right foot, stronger on left foot
2. Hgb 10.5 g and Hct 32%
3. Bowel sounds hypoactive in all quadrants
4. Crackles in the lower bases of the lung

✓✓✓ **Interactive activity:** With a partner, **do the following: (1) select** the **one nursing diagnosis** that is of priority at this time, **(2) provide a rationale** for your selection, and **(3) list the nursing interventions** that assist to meet the needs of the patient.

All of the following nursing diagnoses may apply to Mrs. T:

Acute pain; Risk for infection; Risk for impaired skin integrity; Impaired urinary elimination, Impaired gas exchange, Fatigue, Impaired physical mobility, Ineffective tissue perfusion

Nursing Diagnosis	Rationale	Nursing Interventions
		1. 2. 3.

✓✓✓ On the second post-op day Mrs. T is still very confused and is trying to get OOB. She has bilateral scattered crackles in the lungs, SOB on exertion, R. 32, and a nonproductive cough.

Instructions: Based on the situation above, identify and write the **priority problem** in the box below. Then, starting with the small box labeled **#1 prioritize** the **nursing interventions** for this situation and **identify** your plan for follow-up care for Mrs. T.

NURSING INTERVENTIONS

A. Take vital signs

B. Check O_2 saturation

C. Stay with patient

D. Enc. incentive spirometer hourly

E. Call physician

F. Enc. fluids

DECISION-MAKING DIAGRAM

New Action Plan

#1 #2 #3 #4 #5 #6

Priority Problem

NOTES ______________________

Applying Critical Thinking Skills to Test Questions

INSTRUCTIONS: Circle the one best answer for each test question. Write your rationale for selecting the answer. To enhance your learning and test-taking skill, discuss your answer and rationale with a partner. The answer and the rationale can be found on the back of this page.

1. The nurse is caring for an 82-year-old client who is 1 day post-op left hip replacement. The client has a primary IV infusing at 100 cc/hr, a patient-controlled analgesic device, and a urinary catheter. After assessing the client, the nurse determines that the client is pleasant, cooperative, but forgetful. In the afternoon, the nurse notes that the client has become increasingly restless in the afternoon. It is most important of the nurse to
   a. apply soft restraints.
   b. notify the physician.
   c. check the patient-controlled analgesic device
   d. assess the client's past medical history for dementia.

   Rationale: ____

2. The nurse is delegating the care of a 79-year-old client 2 days post-op hip replacement to a nursing assistant who routinely works on a post-partum unit. Which instruction, given to the nursing assistant, is of priority initially?
   a. Have the client cough and deep breathe q2h.
   b. Total the intake and output at 1400.
   c. Use a fracture bedpan on the client.
   d. Wash the client's skin with a mild soap.

   Rationale: ____

3. The nurse is assisting a client get out of a chair after having a right hip replacement 3 days ago. The client suddenly complains of pain and tells the nurse that it hurts too much to walk. Which nursing intervention is of priority?
   a. Encourage the client to put most of the weight on the left leg.
   b. Support the client's right side as the client is asked to stand up.
   c. Assess the client's right hip and leg.
   d. Administer pain medication.

   Rationale: ____

Applying Critical Thinking Skills to Test Questions

HELPFUL HINTS: Read all test questions carefully. Identify key words in the question that will guide you in answering the question. In these test questions the **key words** to consider are **"most important," "priority initially,"** and **"priority."** Compare your rationale with the one in the test question.

1. The nurse is caring for an 82-year-old client who is 1 day post-op left hip replacement. The client has a primary IV infusing at 100 cc/hr, a patient-controlled analgesic device, and a urinary catheter. After assessing the client, the nurse determines that the client is pleasant, cooperative, but forgetful. In the afternoon, the nurse notes that the client has become increasingly restless in the afternoon. It is most important of the nurse to
   a. apply soft restraints.
   b. notify the physician.
   (c.) check the patient-controlled analgesic device
   d. assess the client's past medical history for dementia.

   Rationale: **(C) is the answer. Pain may be a contributing factor to the client's restlessness. The patient-controlled analgesic device should be checked to see if the client has used it to control the pain. Options (a), (b), and (d) are not appropriate interventions.**

2. The nurse is delegating the care of a 79-year-old client 2 days post-op hip replacement to a nursing assistant who routinely works on a post-partum unit. Which instruction, given to the nursing assistant, is of priority initially?
   a. Have the client cough and deep breathe q2h.
   b. Total the intake and output at 1400.
   (c.) Use a fracture bedpan on the client.
   d. Wash the client's skin with a mild soap.

   Rationale: **(C) is the answer. A fractured bedpan will minimize putting stress on the hip area and preventing hip dislocation. Options (a), (b), and (d) are important, but instructing a new nursing assistant on how to prevent complications on an unfamiliar unit is of priority.**

3. The nurse is assisting a client get out of a chair after having a right hip replacement 3 days ago. The client suddenly complains of pain and tells the nurse that it hurts too much to walk. Which nursing intervention is of priority?
   a. Encourage the client to put most of the weight on the left leg.
   b. Support the client's right side as the client is asked to stand up.
   (c.) Assess the client's right hip and leg.
   d. Administer pain medication.

   Rationale: **(C) is the answer. Increased pain may indicate hip dislocation. Options (a), (b), and (d) are good interventions, but the nurse should assess the surgical site before continuing with any other intervention.**

THE PATIENT WITH A FRACTURED TIBIA

Mr. W, 26 years old, was admitted with a left fractured tibia. He was taken to surgery and is now being transferred to the orthopedic unit. He has a long leg cast on the left leg. His post-op orders are transcribed to the nursing care kardex:

VS q4h I & O (✓) Neurovascular cks (circ. movement, sensation, temp) q4h Elevate left leg on (1) pillow	1L D_5W q10h - dc when taking fluids well Teach crutch walking in AM	Diet: Clear liquids → Reg. PRN med: Meperidine 100 mg IM q4h prn pain

You are assigned to Mr. W as he is taken into his room. You note that he is alert, the left leg cast is damp and clean, and an IV is infusing into his right hand.

Instructions: Prioritize the five **nursing interventions** as you would do them to take care of Mr. W. Write a number in the box to identify the order of your interventions (#1 = first intervention, #2 = second intervention, etc.) and state a **rationale** for each intervention.

INTERVENTIONS	PRIORITY #	RATIONALE
◆ Take the vital signs	☐	______________
◆ Neurovascular assessment of both extremities	☐	______________
◆ Assess cast for dryness, signs of drainage, and sharp edges	☐	______________
◆ Use palms of hands to elevate cast on a pillow	☐	______________
◆ Teach isometric exercises	☐	______________

KEY POINTS TO CONSIDER: ______________

____

On the morning of the first post-op day, you note that Mr. W is:

1. Requesting pain med q4h
2. Left pedal pulses present, edema 2+
3. Capillary refill >2 sec, moves left toes
4. Taking fluids and voiding qs
5. MD orders CPK, LDH, and SGOT

✓✓✓ **Interactive activity:** With a partner, **do the following: (1) select** the **one nursing diagnosis** that is of priority at this time, **(2) provide a rationale** for your selection, and **(3) list the nursing interventions** that assist you to meet the needs of the patient.

All of the following nursing diagnoses may apply to Mr. W:

Risk for injury, Deficient knowledge, Risk for infection, Risk for impaired skin integrity, Impaired physical mobility, Fear, Ineffective tissue perfusion, Pain, Activity intolerance, Impaired tissue integrity, Anxiety, Risk for peripheral neurovascular dysfunction

Nursing Diagnosis	Rationale	Nursing Interventions
		1. 2. 3.

✓✓✓ **Mr. W refuses lunch** and you assess:

c/o increased pain, especially with elevation of the leg, numbness and tingling, left pedal pulse weak, cool

Instructions: Based on this new information, identify and write the **priority problem** in the box below. Then, starting with the small box labeled **#1 prioritize** the **nursing interventions** for this situation and **identify** your follow-up action plan for Mr. W.

NURSING INTERVENTIONS

A. Inform RN/MD stat

B. Prepare to have cast bivalved

C. Ensure left extremity is at heart level

D. Monitor left pedal pulse

E. Take the vital signs

F. Stay with patient

DECISION-MAKING DIAGRAM

New Action Plan

#1 #2 #3 #4 #5 #6

Priority Problem

NOTES ____________________

____

THE PATIENT WITH CATARACT SURGERY

Mrs. G, 72 years old, has senile cataracts and has been instilling mydriatic eye drops. Her vision has progressively worsened and she is scheduled today for a right cataract extraction in the outpatient clinic. The MD orders the following pre-op preparation: NPO; instill mydriatic and cycloplegic eye drops 1 hour before surgery; Valium 5 mg po 1 hour before surgery. Mrs. G arrives at the outpatient clinic at 0800 and she is scheduled for surgery at 1000.

Instructions: Prioritize the five **nursing interventions** as you would do them to take care of Mrs. G. Write a number in the box to identify the order of your interventions (#1 = first intervention, #2 = second intervention, etc.) and state a **rationale** for each intervention.

INTERVENTIONS	PRIORITY #	RATIONALE
◆ Provide information regarding pre-op preparation	☐	
◆ Begin to instill ordered eye drops	☐	
◆ Have patient void	☐	
◆ Take the vital signs	☐	
◆ Ensure the surgical consent is signed prior to initiating pre-op preparation	☐	

KEY POINTS TO CONSIDER:

Mrs. G had an intraocular lens implant and is taken to the recovery room. She has an eye patch on her right eye and you assess the following:

1. No c/o pain, P. 88 - B/P 130/82
2. Eye patch clean and dry
3. Readily responds to verbal stimuli

✓✓✓ **Interactive activity:** With a partner, **do the following: (1) select** the **one nursing diagnosis** that is of priority at this time, **(2) provide a rationale** for your selection, and **(3) list the nursing interventions** that assist to meet the needs of the patient.

All of the following nursing diagnoses may apply to Mrs. G:

Risk for injury, Deficient knowledge, Disturbed sensory perception, Fear, Anxiety, Risk for self-care deficit, Risk for infection, Ineffective health maintenance, Impaired home maintenance, Sensory-perceptual alterations: visual

Nursing Diagnosis	Rationale	Nursing Interventions
		1. 2. 3.

✓✓✓ One hour **post-op** you assess Mrs. G and note the following:

c/o right brow pain, anxious, P. 110 - B/P 128/80 coughing and c/o nausea

Instructions: Based on the **post-op** assessment, identify and write the **priority problem** in the box below. Then, starting with the small box labeled **#1 prioritize** the **nursing interventions** for this situation and **identify** your follow-up action plan for Mrs. G.

NURSING INTERVENTIONS

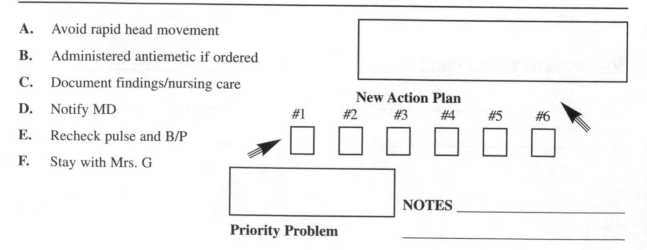

A. Avoid rapid head movement

B. Administered antiemetic if ordered

C. Document findings/nursing care

D. Notify MD

E. Recheck pulse and B/P

F. Stay with Mrs. G

DECISION-MAKING DIAGRAM

New Action Plan

#1 #2 #3 #4 #5 #6

Priority Problem

NOTES ____________________

____

THE PATIENT WITH A SEIZURE DISORDER

Mr. M, 20 years old, fell at home and was brought to the emergency room after it was noticed that he had lost consciousness for a few seconds. In the emergency room he indicated that he did not remember falling. His family history is significant for seizure disorders. Diagnostic studies were ordered and included an EEG, MRI, serum fasting blood sugar, CBC, BUN, and UA drug screening. He was just transferred to the neurological unit from the emergency room. The current MD orders include: seizure precautions, bed rest, soft diet, saline lock, vital signs, and neuro checks q4h.

Instructions: Prioritize the following **nursing interventions** as you would do them to initially take care of Mr. M. Write a number in the box to identify the order of your interventions (#1 = first intervention, #2 = second intervention, etc.) and state a **rationale** for each intervention.

INTERVENTIONS	PRIORITY #	RATIONALE
◆ Orient Mr. M to his room	☐	
◆ Assess neurological status	☐	
◆ Implement seizure precautions	☐	
◆ Obtain admitting history	☐	
◆ Inform of pertinent MD orders	☐	

KEY POINTS TO CONSIDER:

Mr. M is diagnosed with a seizure disorder and is started on Depakote. In speaking with Mr. M you gather the following:

1. Mr. M says that he has had similar episodes but never told anyone.
2. He remembers seeing "spots" before the episode.
3. No one in his family talked much about the relative who had seizures.

✓✓✓ **Interactive activity:** With a partner, **do the following: (1) select** the **one nursing diagnosis** that is of priority at this time, **(2) provide a rationale** for your selection, and **(3) list the nursing interventions** that assist you to meet the needs of the patient.

All of the following nursing diagnoses may apply to Mr. M:

Ineffective coping, Ineffective airway clearance, Risk for injury, Deficient knowledge, Disturbed self-concept, Social isolation, Fear, Anxiety, Disturbed thought processes, Risk for aspiration

Nursing Diagnosis	Rationale	Nursing Interventions
		1. 2. 3.

✓✓✓ Several hours after admission, you hear a "cry" coming from Mr. M's room. You assess the following as you walk into the room:

Tonic-clonic movements of the body, loss of consciousness, excessive salivation, some cyanosis, urinary incontinence, teeth clenched with cessation of tonic-clonic movements after 3 min.

Instructions: Based on the situation above, identify and write the **priority problem** in the box below. Then, starting with the small box labeled **#1 prioritize** the **nursing interventions** for this situation and identify your follow-up action plan for Mr. M.

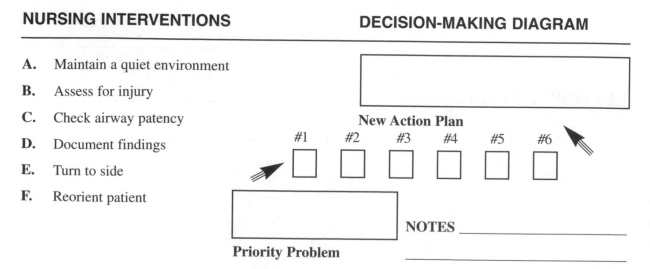

NURSING INTERVENTIONS

A. Maintain a quiet environment

B. Assess for injury

C. Check airway patency

D. Document findings

E. Turn to side

F. Reorient patient

DECISION-MAKING DIAGRAM

New Action Plan

#1 #2 #3 #4 #5 #6

Priority Problem

NOTES ____________________

____

Applying Critical Thinking Skills to Test Questions

INSTRUCTIONS: Circle the one best answer for each test question. Write your rationale for selecting the answer. To enhance your learning and test-taking skill, discuss your answer and rationale with a partner. The answer and the rationale can be found on the back of this page.

1. The nurse documents the following after observing a client have a tonic-clonic seizure: "0930 Found client having jerky, involuntary movements of upper and lower extremities lasting 2 minutes, frothy saliva oozing from mouth, incontinent of urine." Which statement best describes the nurse's charting? The charting
   a. is appropriate and describes the observations seen.
   b. should include the client's response and nursing interventions.
   c. should just indicate that the client had a tonic-clonic seizure.
   d. is lacking whether the client had an aura experience prior to the seizure.

   Rationale: ______________________________

2. The nurse admits a client who is having uncontrolled generalized tonic-clonic seizures. In planning for potential complications, which nursing intervention is of priority?
   a. Have a tongue blade next to the client's bed.
   b. Have suction equipment available.
   c. Maintain side rails up at all times.
   d. Maintain a quiet environment.

   Rationale: ______________________________

3. The nurse is caring for a client who is on phenytoin (Dilantin) 200 mg po tid and phenobarbital 20 mg po tid. Which assessment finding is most indicative of a common drug side effect?
   a. Gums red and swollen
   b. Complaints of constipation
   c. Respiratory depression
   d. Skin rash

   Rationale: ______________________________

Applying Critical Thinking Skills to Test Questions

HELPFUL HINTS: Read all test questions carefully. Identify key words in the question that will guide you in answering the question. In these test questions the **key words** to consider are **"best," "priority,"** and **"most indicative."** Compare your rationale with the one in the test question.

1. The nurse documents the following after observing a client have a tonic-clonic seizure: "0930 Found client having jerky, involuntary movements of upper and lower extremities lasting 2 minutes, frothy saliva oozing from mouth, incontinent of urine." Which statement best describes the nurse's charting? The charting
   a. is appropriate and describes the observations seen.
   (b.) should include the client's response and nursing interventions.
   c. should just indicate that the client had a tonic-clonic seizure.
   d. is lacking whether the client had an aura experience prior to the seizure.

   Rationale: **(B) is the answer. Charting should include what is observed, the nursing interventions, and the client's response/reaction. Options (a), (c), and (d) do not include all of the components necessary for legal documentation.**

2. The nurse admits a client who is having uncontrolled generalized tonic-clonic seizures. In planning for potential complications, which nursing intervention is of priority?
   a. Have a tongue blade next to the client's bed.
   (b.) Have suction equipment available.
   c. Maintain side rails up at all times.
   d. Maintain a quiet environment.

   Rationale: **(B) is the answer. Suction equipment is necessary to clear oral secretions after the seizure and prevent aspiration. Options (c) and (d) are important, but preventing aspiration is of priority. Option (a) is not a current intervention.**

3. The nurse is caring for a client who is on phenytoin (Dilantin) 200 mg po tid and phenobarbital 20 mg po tid. Which assessment finding is most indicative of a common drug side effect?
   (a.) Gums red and swollen
   b. Complaints of constipation
   c. Respiratory depression
   d. Skin rash

   Rationale: **(A) is the answer. Gingival hyperplasia is a common side effect seen with the administration of phenytoin. Meticulous oral hygiene is an important intervention. Option (b) is not a common side effect. Option (c) is a toxic reaction to phenobarbital, and option (d) is a toxic reaction to phenytoin.**

THE PATIENT WITH A DNR ORDER

Mr. B, 83 years old, has terminal esophageal cancer. The following pertinent information is found in the nursing care rand:

Activity: Bed rest Vital signs: q4h O_2 sats: q4h Lives with son Hospital Day: #4	PEG tube insertion: 3 days ago Formula full strength – 50 ml/hr Ck residual q4h, if > 100 ml hold feeding for 1 hour MS 2 mg IV q2h prn pain	IV: D_5/0.45 NS q12h Urinary catheter inserted on admission I & O q8h Code Status: No code

The 7:00 AM report indicates that his current respirations are 10 and he last received MS at 6:00 AM. Residual at that time was 125 ml; tube feeding was stopped. IV has 200 ml left.

Instructions: Prioritize the five **nursing interventions** as you would do them to initially take care of Mr. B. Write a number in the box to identify the order of your interventions (#1= first intervention, #2= second intervention, etc.) and state a **rationale** for each intervention.

INTERVENTIONS	PRIORITY #	RATIONALE
◆ Assess PEG tube residual	☐	
◆ Take the vital signs	☐	
◆ Assess IV site and IV fluid level	☐	
◆ Perform a body system's assessment	☐	
◆ Assess O_2 saturation level	☐	

KEY POINTS TO CONSIDER:

At 11:00 AM Mr. B manifested the following signs and symptoms:

1. VS: P. 76 - R.14 - B/P 118/64
2. Responds appropriately, but is weak and lethargic
3. Urine is dark yellow; output 125 cc since 7:00 AM
4. SOB when turning; irregular breathing pattern

✓✓✓ **Interactive activity:** With a partner, **do the following: (1) select** the **one nursing diagnosis** that is of priority at this time, **(2) provide a rationale** for your selection, and **(3) list the nursing interventions** that assist to meet the needs of the patient.

All of the following nursing diagnoses may apply to Mr. B:

Risk for infection, Pain, Anxiety, Impaired gas exchange, Imbalanced nutrition: less than body requirements, Risk for deficient fluid volume, Risk for impaired skin integrity, Ineffective tissue perfusion, Activity intolerance, Powerlessness, Social isolation

Nursing Diagnosis	Rationale	Nursing Interventions
		1. 2. 3.

✓✓✓ At **2:00 PM** Mr. B is unresponsive to verbal stimuli. You assessed:

VS: P. 36 - R. 9 - B/P 80/50. Urine output unchanged since 11:00 AM. Lower extremities cool with cyanosis.

Instructions: Based on the **2:00 PM** assessment, identify and write the **priority problem** in the box below. Then, starting with the small box labeled **#1 prioritize** the **nursing interventions** for this situation and **identify** your plan for follow-up care for Mr. B.

NURSING INTERVENTIONS

A. Monitor vital signs
B. Check NCP for religious/cultural requests
C. Report findings to RN
D. Notify relatives
E. Provide comfort measures
F. Document findings

DECISION-MAKING DIAGRAM

New Action Plan

#1 #2 #3 #4 #5 #6

Priority Problem

NOTES ______________________

____

LEGAL CONSIDERATIONS

Mrs. L is 1 day post-op total abdominal hysterectomy. She is 42 years old. Demerol 75 mg is ordered IM q3h prn pain. She is on a clear liquid diet and has not voided since the urinary catheter was removed at noon. She is ambulating with assistance to the bathroom. The abdominal dressing is stained with dried dark red drainage. Vital signs at noon are T. 99° F - P. 82 - R. 22 - B/P 130/76. Fine crackles are audible in the lower bases of the lung fields. It is 4:00 PM and she is requesting pain medication. Her last pain shot was administered at 2:00 PM. An incentive spirometer is at the bedside.

Instructions: Prioritize the following **nursing interventions** as you, the nurse, would do them to initially take care of Mrs. L. Write a number in the box to identify the order of your interventions (#1 = first intervention, #2 = second intervention, etc.) and state a **rationale** for each intervention.

INTERVENTIONS	PRIORITY #	RATIONALE
◆ Inform Mrs. L that the pain medication is not due for another hour	☐	
◆ Cough and deep breathe; demonstrate abdominal splinting; use incentive spirometer q1h	☐	
◆ Ambulate to the bathroom	☐	
◆ Take the vitals signs	☐	
◆ Assess abdomen and surgical dressing	☐	

KEY POINTS TO CONSIDER: ______

Mrs. L voids 400 cc after ambulating to the bathroom and states that she feels much better. She relates the following to you:

1. Her mother had a hysterectomy, but died 10 days after from surgical complications.
2. She is glad that she does not have to worry about irregular periods any more.
3. She fully trusts her doctor but wonders whether the right thing was done.
4. She lives alone.

✓✓✓ **Interactive activity:** With a partner, **do the following: (1) select** the **one nursing diagnosis** that is of priority at this time, **(2) provide a rationale** for your selection, and **(3) list the nursing interventions** that assist to meet the needs of the patient.

All of the following nursing diagnoses may apply to Mrs. L:

Risk for infection, Pain, Anxiety, Ineffective breathing pattern, Imbalanced nutrition: less than body requirements, Disturbed body image, Sexual dysfunction, Impaired skin integrity, Risk for activity intolerance, Deficient knowledge

Nursing Diagnosis	Rationale	Nursing Interventions
		1. 2. 3.

✓✓✓ At 6:00 PM Mrs. L states that she is having pain. In fact on a scale from 1-10, Mrs. L's pain is an 8. She has not received any pain medication since 2:00 PM.

You take out an ampule labeled Demerol 100 mg/ml and administer 1 ml.
Mrs. L asks whether the 75 mg of Demerol would help her since it did not help her before.

Instructions: Based on the situation above, identify and write the **priority problem** in the box below. Then, starting with the small box labeled **#1 prioritize** the **nursing interventions** for this situation and **identify** your follow-up action plan for Mrs. L.

NURSING INTERVENTIONS

A. Tell the patient you administered 100 mg of Demerol
B. Document drug and amount given
C. Monitor vital signs
D. Fill out an incident report
E. Notify your instructor
F. Notify physician

DECISION-MAKING DIAGRAM

New Action Plan

#1 #2 #3 #4 #5 #6

Priority Problem

NOTES ______________________

____

SECTION THREE

Applying the Critical Thinking Model

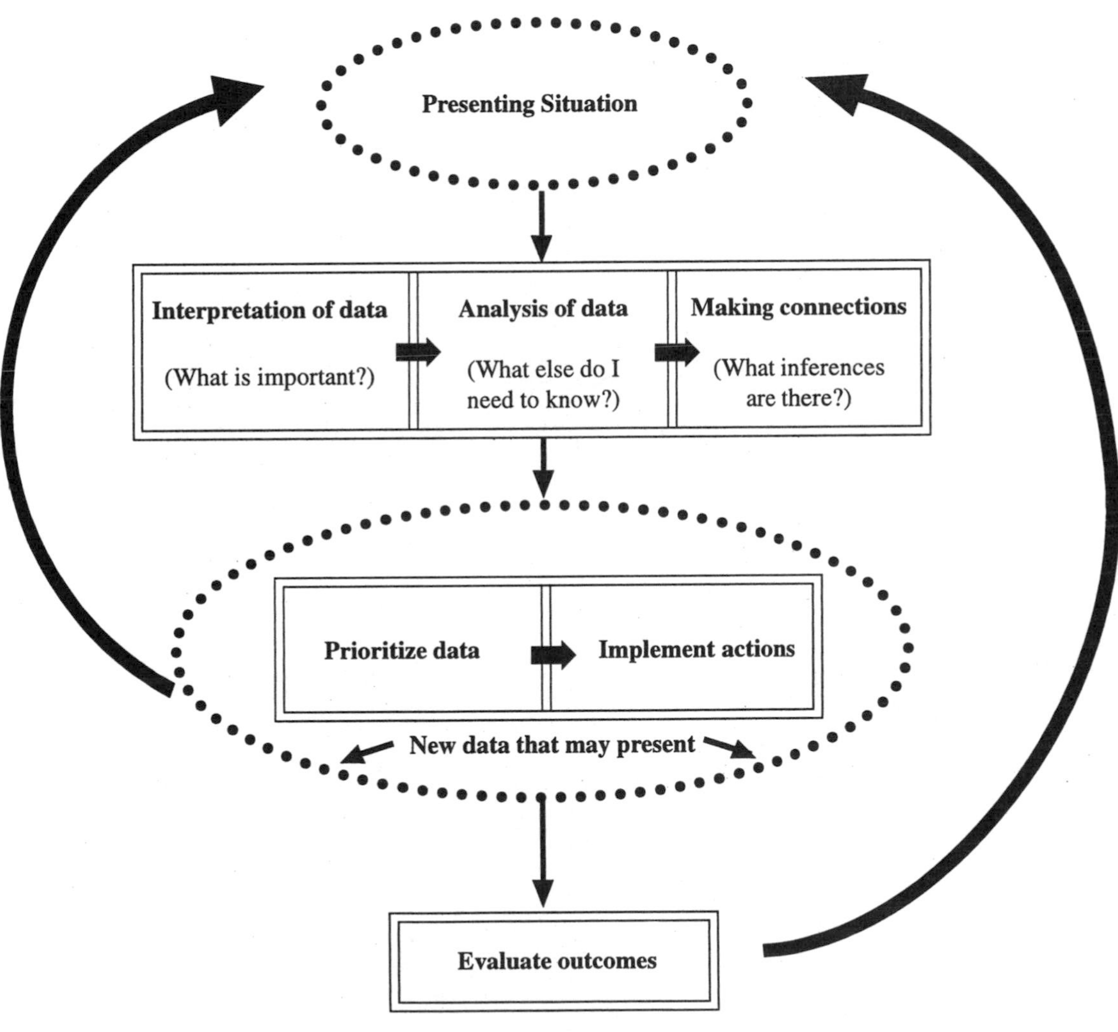

CLINICAL SITUATION - # 1

Intershift taped report at 0700:

"Mr. A, 72 years old, is 2 days post-op small bowel resection. His N/G tube is connected to low wall suction and is draining dark brown fluid. Vital signs at 0600: T. 99.6° F - P. 90 - R. 28 - B/P 160/94. IV D_5/0.45 NS with 20 mEq KCl infusing at 125 cc into the right forearm. He is using the PCA machine. He slept most of the night and is now sitting in a chair. SOB was noted when he was transferred to the chair. There are 300 cc left in the IV."

Mr. A's current **flow charts** contain the following information:

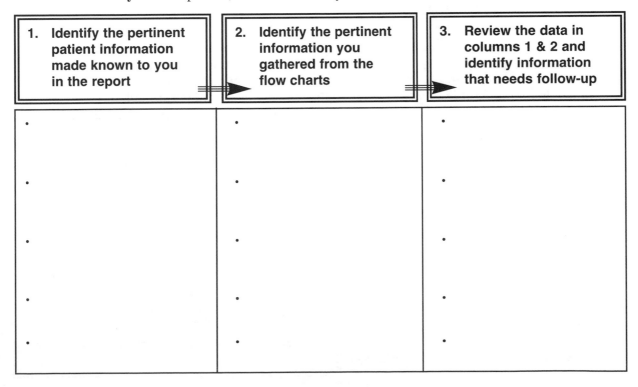

Medication Record

Routine	Time Due
Lanoxin 0.25 mg IV qd	0900
Lasix 20 mg IVP qd	0900
Timolol 0.25% gtt i̅ OU BID	1000
Protonix 40 mg IVPB qd	1000
Gentamicin 80 mg IVPB q8h	1400
PRN	
Phenergan 25 mg IV/IM q4h prn N/V	
PCA (morphine sulfate - 1mg/hr)	

Intake and Output Record

Night Shift @ 0600

Intake			Output		
P.O.	=	0	UA void	=	0
			Foley	=	200
IV	=	1000	N/G	=	600
IVPB	=	100			

Interactive activity: With a partner, use the case study and the flow charts to:

1. Identify the pertinent patient information made known to you in the report	2. Identify the pertinent information you gathered from the flow charts	3. Review the data in columns 1 & 2 and identify information that needs follow-up
•	•	•
•	•	•
•	•	•
•	•	•
•	•	•

It is 0730 as you leave the report room, **prioritize** your plan of care for the morning:

Time	Plan of Nursing Care

➤ **1200 nursing assessment:** Oriented x3, skin WNL, capillary refill < 3 sec., turgor good, mucous membranes moist, pinkish, T. 99° F - P. 88 slightly irregular - R. 24 - B/P 164/94. N/G draining brownish fluid 100 cc since 0800. Bowel sounds present x4, abd. soft. Foley catheter draining clear yellow urine.

Mr. A has minimal complaints and is visited by the physician at 1200. The physician leaves the following orders:

Remove Foley now
Enc. incentive spirometer q1h x10
Discontinue N/G tube
DC Lasix
Lanoxin 0.25 mg po qd
Hgb & Hct today
Clear liquid diet

1. Identify the nursing interventions that require immediate follow-up	2. Identify the nursing actions that you can delegate/assign to unlicensed personnel

For each of the following **nursing interventions**, write an **expected patient outcome**:

1. Foley removed at 1300 ⟹
2. Incentive spirometer q1h x10 ⟹

CLINICAL SITUATION - # 2

Intershift taped report at 7:00 AM:

"The patient is 43 years old and was admitted 2 nights ago after experiencing GI bleed. He is NPO and has an N/G tube connected to continuous suction. The N/G has drained 100 cc of dark reddish drainage. Vital signs at 6:00 AM are T. 97.4° F - P. 96 - R. 18 - B/P 130/86. A unit of whole blood is infusing and should be complete by 9:00 AM. His current Hgb is 8.6. He does have a history of ETOH abuse and has been more restless this morning."

The patient's current **flow charts** contain the following information:

Patient Care Kardex

IV: D_5/0.9 NS c̄ 10cc MVI @ 100 cc/hr

IV site: #18 g LFA; saline lock RFA#20 g

Give two units of whole blood today ☑ ☐
H & H in the AM

Routine Medication:
Mylanta 30 cc q4h/NG (clamp tube for 30min p̄ administration)
Famotidine 20 mg q12h 10-10

Intake and Output Record

Night Shift @ 0600

Intake		**Output**	
P.O.	= 0	UA void	= 525
		N/G	= 100
IV	= 600		
0.9NS	= 50		
Transfusion	= 50		

Interactive activity: With a partner, **use the case study and the flow charts** to:

1. Identify the pertinent patient information made known to you in the report	2. Identify the pertinent information you gathered from the flow charts	3. Review the data in columns 1 & 2 and identify information that needs follow-up
•	•	•
•	•	•
•	•	•
•	•	•
•	•	•
•		
•		
•		

It is 7:30 AM as you leave the report room, **prioritize** your plan of care for the morning:

Time	Plan of Nursing Care

➤ **10:00 AM nursing assessment:** Anxious, restless, pulled out N/G tube. Physician called. Wrist restraints applied. VS: P. 100 - R. 26 - B/P 146/90. Vomited 20 cc bright red fluid. Bowel sounds present x4, abd. soft. Transfusion #2 infusing at 25 gtt/min.

The physician calls back and gives the following telephone orders:

Wrist and vest posey restraints prn
Oxygen at 2L/min/NP
Reinsert NG tube
ABG, serum electrolytes Mg^{++}, BS, H & H
VS and neuro checks q2h
Librium 50 mg IM q3h prn restlessness
Phenergan 25 mg IM q4h prn N/V

1. Identify the nursing interventions that require immediate follow-up	2. Identify the nursing actions that you can delegate/assign to unlicensed personnel

For each of the following **nursing interventions**, write **expected patient outcomes:**

1. Application of wrist and vest posey ⟹

2. Librium 50 mg IM ⟹

CLINICAL SITUATION - # 3

Intershift taped report at 1600:

"The patient was admitted today with dehydration. She is 88 years old and has a Stage IV pressure ulcer on her sacrum. A wet-to-dry dressing was applied. A pressure ulcer with eschar is on her left heel. She weighs 90 lb and she refused her lunch. An IV was started at 1400. You have 750 cc credit. She is a sweet little lady, quiet, and at times forgetful. Her admission lab results just came in, her Hgb is 9.6, Hct 27, WBC 11,000, and K+ 4.5. I have not called the physician."

The patient's current **flow charts** contain the following information:

Patient Care Kardex

VS q4h — Diet: Pureed
HOH
Siderails ↑ at all times
W-D Drsg $\bar{c}$ 0.9 NS 0600-1400-2200

IV: D_5/0.9 NS at 75 cc/hr
IV site: R hand #24 g cannula

Medication: Colace 100 mg qd

NO CODE

Intake and Output Record

Day Shift - 8 hour

Intake			Output
P.O.	=	50	UA = inc x2
IV	=	250	

Interactive activity: With a partner, **use the case study and the flow charts** to:

1. Identify the pertinent patient information made known to you in the report	2. Identify the pertinent information you gathered from the flow charts	3. Review the data in columns 1 & 2 and identify information that needs follow-up
•	•	•
•	•	•
•	•	•
•	•	•
•	•	•
	•	
	•	

It is 1630 as you leave the report room, **prioritize** your plan of care for the next 4 hours:

Time	Plan of Nursing Care

➢ **At 2000** the nursing assistant reports that the patient is restless and trying to get out of bed. You document the following assessment: Speech incoherent, skin warm, flushed. VS: T. 101° F - P. 92 - R. 24 - B/P 108/60. Incontinent of dark-colored urine with strong odor. Physician called. The following telephone orders are given:

Catheterize for post-residual urine
VS q2h, I & O
Tylenol 325 mg po q4h prn T. > 100.4° F
Vest posey restraint prn
Enc. fluid intake
Rocephin 1 g IVPB qd

1. Identify the nursing interventions that require immediate follow-up	2. Identify the nursing actions that you can delegate/assign to unlicensed personnel

For the following **nursing intervention**, write an **expected patient outcome**:

1. Monitor I & O q8h ⟹

CLINICAL SITUATION - # 4

Intershift taped report at 2300:

"The patient was admitted with a fractured right tibia and is 1 day post-op. He has a cast on. He has been quiet most of the evening. He just started coughing and is experiencing some SOB. He says he has a history of asthma and that he gets this way every now and then. I did not detect any wheezing. Vital signs are T. 98.8° F - P. 90 - R. 28 - B/P 140/88. Circulation, movement, and sensation are WNL in the right leg."

The patient's current **flow charts** contain the following information:

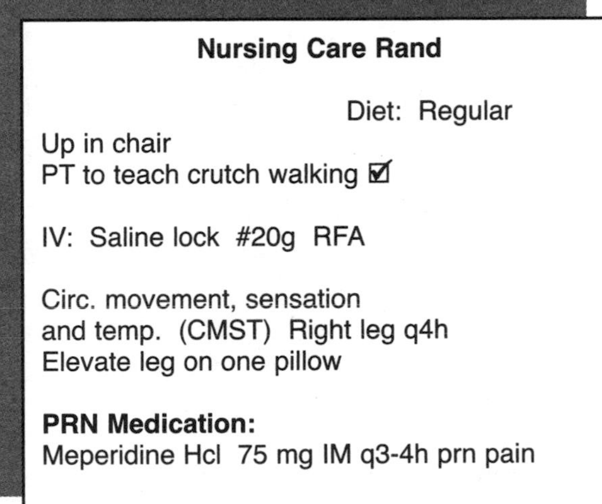

Nursing Care Rand

Diet: Regular

Up in chair
PT to teach crutch walking ☑

IV: Saline lock #20g RFA

Circ. movement, sensation
and temp. (CMST) Right leg q4h
Elevate leg on one pillow

PRN Medication:
Meperidine Hcl 75 mg IM q3-4h prn pain

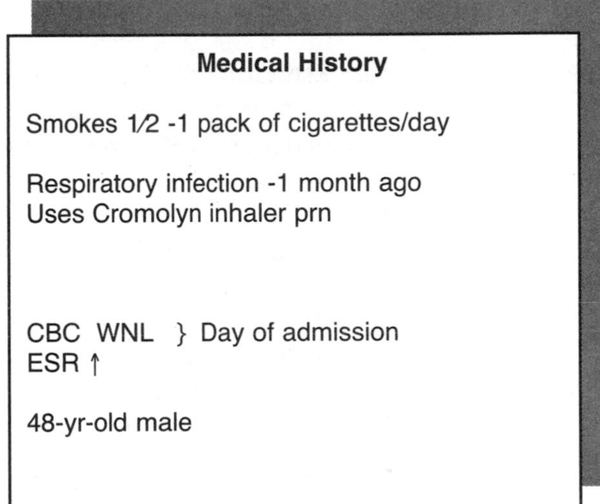

Medical History

Smokes 1/2 -1 pack of cigarettes/day

Respiratory infection -1 month ago
Uses Cromolyn inhaler prn

CBC WNL } Day of admission
ESR ↑

48-yr-old male

Interactive activity: With a partner, **use the case study and the flow charts** to:

1. Identify the pertinent patient information made known to you in the report	2. Identify the pertinent information you gathered from the flow charts	3. Review the data in columns 1 & 2 and identify information that needs follow-up
•	•	•
•	•	•
•	•	•
•	•	•
•	•	•
•	•	
•		

It is 2330 as you leave the report room, **prioritize** your plan of care for the next 3 hours:

Time	Plan of Nursing Care

➤ **0200 nursing assessment:** The patient is beginning to cough more frequently; c/o chest tightness. Respiratory assessment indicates inspiratory and expiratory wheezes in bilateral lungs. You call the physician and obtain the following telephone orders:

IV D_5/0.9 NS at 125 cc/hr
Oxygen at 2 L/NP
Ventolin inhaler 2 puffs q4h
Alupent nebulizer treatment q3h
ABG, sputum for eosinophils
Solu-medrol 125 mg IVP q6h
Check oxygen saturation with pulse oximeter q2h
Call physician with ABG results

1. Identify the nursing interventions that require immediate follow-up	2. Identify the nursing actions that you can delegate/assign to unlicensed personnel

For each of the following **nursing interventions**, write an **expected patient outcome**:

1. Alupent treatment q3h ⟹
2. Solu-medrol 125 mg IVP ⟹

CLINICAL SITUATION - # 5

Intershift taped report at 3:00 PM:

"Mrs. C, 42 years old, was admitted earlier today with acute pancreatitis. She had mid-epigastric pain with nausea and vomiting on admission. Her latest vitals signs are T. 38° C - P. 108 - R. 26 - B/P 110/60. Bowel sounds are hypoactive. I medicated her at 2:00 PM. A central line was inserted, you have 800 cc left in the IV. The N/G is draining brownish fluid. She needs to have the urinary catheter inserted."

Mrs. C's current **flow charts** contain the following information:

Patient Care Kardex

VS: q4hrs Diet: NPO
O_2 @ 3 L/NP
Pulse oximetry q4h

IV: D_5W @125 cc/hr
Right central line
N/G tube to low con't suction ☑
Urinary catheter inserted ☐

ABG in am ☐
K^+, Na^+, Cl^-, CO_2, Mg^{2+}, Ca^{++} in AM ☐
Abd CT scan @ 6 PM today

Routine Medication:
Famotidine 20 mg q12h 10-10

PRN Medication:
Meperidine 75 mg IM q3h prn pain

Admission Lab Data

Se Amylase	350 units/L
Se Lipase	260 units/L
Hgb	11.6 g/dl
Hct	32%
WBC	18,000/mm^3
LDH	300 units/L
AST	80 units/L
BS	200 mg/dl

Interactive activity: With a partner, **use the case study and the flow charts** to:

1. Identify the pertinent patient information made known to you in the report	2. Identify the pertinent information you gathered from the flow charts	3. Review the data in columns 1 & 2 and identify information that needs follow-up
•	•	•
•	•	•
•	•	•
•	•	•
•	•	•
•	•	•

It is 4:00 PM, **prioritize** your plan of care for the next 3 hours:

Time	Plan of Nursing Care

➢ At 8:30 PM the nursing assistant informs you that Mrs. C is complaining of pain and is restless. You note that she has not had a pain shot in the last 3 hours. You walk into the room to assess her and to give her a meperidine injection. She turns over quickly and pulls out the central line.

1. Identify the nursing interventions that you would implement immediately at the bedside	2. Identify the follow-up nursing actions. Document the incident in the nurse's notes.

Nurse's Notes

For the following **nursing intervention**, write the **expected patient outcome**:

1. Call physician regarding abnormal lab values ⟹

CLINICAL SITUATION - # 6

Intershift taped report at 8:00 AM:

"The patient is a young man who was transferred from the ICU yesterday. He was in a MVA 14 days ago. He had some head trauma and subsequent evacuation of a subdural hematoma. He is unconscious, unresponsive to painful stimuli, and flaccid. Pupils sluggish. He has several abrasions on his face and several bruised areas on his shoulders and chest from the accident. Vital signs are T 97.8° F - P. 94 - R. 24 - B/P 124/80. Mother at bedside; she questions everything you do."

The patient's current **flow charts** contain the following information:

Nursing Care Rand

Suction prn — Diet: NPO
VS & Neuro checks q4h
Seizure precautions — Foley ☑
HOB ↑ 30° at all times — I & O
LBM: ______ PEG tube clamped
IV: D_5/0.9% NS @ 100 cc/ hr via ® central line
Fingerstick BS q6h 12-6-12-6

Routine Medication:
Decadron 4 mg IVP q6h 10-4-10-4
Dulcolax supp. prn

Medical History

18-year-old high school student involved in a MVA in which he was the driver. Passenger in the car died from the injuries.
Pt. unconscious on arrival to the ER.

Drug use: Family not aware of any use. Blood alcohol level on admission 0.16%

Family wants to continue all possible treatment. Not willing to discuss code status at this time.

Interactive activity: With a partner, **use the case study and the flow charts** to:

1. Identify the pertinent patient information made known to you in the report →	2. Identify the pertinent information you gathered from the flow charts →	3. Review the data in columns 1 & 2 and identify information that needs follow-up
•	•	•
•	•	•
•	•	•
•	•	•
•	•	•
•	•	•
•	•	•

It is 8:30 AM as you leave the report room, **prioritize** your plan of care for the next 3 hours:

Time	Plan of Nursing Care

➤ **2:00 PM nursing assessment:** Pupil R • L • R. 12 Cheyne-Stokes. Pulse 80, B/P 150/80. Skin warm, jerky movements of the upper extremity noted. The physician writes the following orders:

Oxygen at 2 L/min/NP
Check oxygen saturation q1h
Vital signs q1h
CT scan stat
ABGs stat

1. Identify the nursing interventions that require immediate follow-up	2. Identify the nursing actions that you can delegate/assign to unlicensed personnel

For each of the following **nursing interventions**, write an **expected patient outcome**:

1. Oxygen 2 L/NP ⟹ [ ]
2. Seizure precautions ⟹ [ ]

CLINICAL SITUATION - # 7

Intershift taped report at 8:00 AM:

"The patient is 52 years old and has bone cancer. She has been requesting pain medication every 2 hours. I gave her MS 2 mg this morning at 6:30 AM. Her respirations have gone down to 10 during the night. She does not want to be turned. A urinary catheter was inserted in the evening shift. She is a no code. A family member spent the night with her. Latest vital signs at 6:00 AM are, T. 97° F - P. 66 - R. 12 - B/P 128/60."

The patient's current **flow charts** contain the following information:

Patient Care Kardex

Diet: DAT

VS q4hrs

Foley ☑

Comfort measures
I & O

IV: Saline lock

LBM: inc. x1 sml

PRN Medication:
MS 2 mg IV q2h prn
MS 4 mg IV q2h prn if not relieved with MS 2 mg

No code

Nurse's Notes

Night shift

11:00 PM Awake, responds when spoken to. c/o generalized pain, refuses to be turned. Medicated with MS 2 mg IV. ——C. Todd RN

11:30 Resp 10, moans when touched, taking sips of water. Mouth care given. C. Todd RN

12:00 AM Moaning. Daughter upset, crying states is afraid that mother is going to die. Referral to pastoral care given. C. Todd RN

1:00 MS 2 mg given IV, lethargic, arouseable resp. 10, p. 60 B/P 110/58. ——C. Todd RN

4:30 Pain med. given ——C. Todd RN

5:00 Resting ——C. Todd RN

6:00 Lethargic but arousable ——C. Todd RN

Interactive activity: With a partner, **use the case study and the flow charts** to:

1. Identify the pertinent patient information made known to you in the report	2. Identify the pertinent information you gathered from the flow charts	3. Review the data in columns 1 & 2 and identify information that needs follow-up
•	•	•
•	•	•
•	•	•
•	•	
•	•	
•		
•		

It is 8:30 AM as you leave the report room, **prioritize** your plan of care for the next 3 hours:

Time	Plan of Nursing Care

➤ **At 12:30 PM** you return from lunch to learn that the nursing assistant was unable to obtain a pulse on the patient. You assess the following: Unresponsive, skin cool, legs pale with mottling. Pulse not palpable, no apical or B/P audible. Family with patient. Physician contacted and pronounced patient.

Family is making arrangements for a mortuary to pick up the patient within the hour.

1. Identify the nursing interventions that require immediate follow-up	2. Identify the nursing actions that you can delegate/assign to unlicensed personnel

For each of the following **nursing interventions**, write an **expected patient outcome**:

1. Provide post-mortem care ⟹ ______

2. Speak with family ⟹ ______

CLINICAL SITUATION - # 8

Intershift taped report at 7:00 AM:

"Mrs. F, 79 years old, was in a motor vehicle accident 2 days ago in which she fractured her arm. Her right arm is in a cast, circulation, movement, and sensation are fine. She is scheduled to go home this morning. She slept fine and was medicated for pain once during the night with relief."

"**At 7:30 AM**, as you are coming out of report, the night nurse tells you that Mrs. F got up to go to the bathroom and fell coming back to bed. She has a slight nosebleed, was given an icepack and assisted back to bed. The physician was called and informed of her falling. He said he would be in later to see her before discharge."

Mrs. F's current **flow charts** contain the following information:

Nursing Care Rand

VS: qs Diet: DAT

LBM: 1 day ago

Discharge this AM.
Discharge instructions: Office appt. 2 wk
Vicodin tab ī po q4h prn

PRN Medication:
Vicodin tab ī po q4h prn
Benadryl 25 mg p.o. HS prn q4-6h

Nurse's Notes

Night shift
11:00 PM Awake, oriented x3. Skin warm and dry. Pulse 88, slightly irregular, lung sound diminished bilaterally in the lower bases. Enc. to take deep breaths, used inspirometer x5. Right arm with cast, CMS-WNL. Requesting sleeping medication. Benadryl 25mg po given. Side rails up. —— S. Dolle RN
1:30 AM Sleeping —— S. Dolle RN
4:30 AM Awake, requesting pain medication CMS-WNL. Vicodin tab ī given S. Dolle RN
6:00 Resting comfortably. —— S. Dolle RN

Interactive activity: With a partner, **use the case study and the flow charts** to:

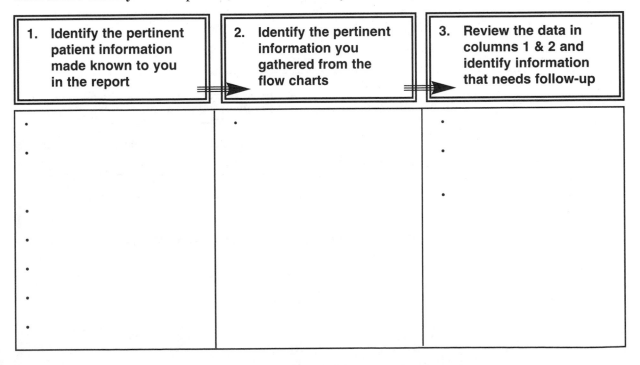

1. Identify the pertinent patient information made known to you in the report	2. Identify the pertinent information you gathered from the flow charts	3. Review the data in columns 1 & 2 and identify information that needs follow-up
• • • • • • •	•	• • •

It is 7:30 AM, **prioritize** your plan of care for the next hour:

Time	Plan of Nursing Care

➤ **At 8:30 AM** you note that Mrs. F is lethargic and very slow to respond to verbal stimuli. Skin is cool with slight cyanosis noted on nailbeds. P. 110 irregular, R. shallow - B/P 90/70, which is lower than her usual of 130/88.

1. Identify the nursing interventions that you would plan to implement immediately	2. Identify the nursing actions that you can delegate/assign to unlicensed personnel

For each of the following **nursing interventions**, write an **expected patient outcome**:

1. Oxygen at 2 L/min/NP ➡ ____________________

2. Insert saline lock ➡ ____________________

CLINICAL SITUATION - # 9

Intershift taped report at 0700:

You are assigned to the following two patients:
"Mrs. A is 52 years old and has diabetes and hypertension. She is in for a pressure ulcer on her right heel. She is on bed rest with the right leg elevated and she only has BRP. There is a wet-to-dry dressing change due at 10. Her latest B/P is 170/108."

"Mrs. C is 73 years old and was admitted with dehydration 3 days ago. She is eating and voiding normally. There is a possibility that she is going home today. I removed her saline lock; there was some redness at the site. She is not on any IV meds, so I decided not to restart. She says that she is going home late this afternoon, although there is no order. Her morning vital signs are T. 97° F - P. 82 - R. 8 - B/P 130/90."

Mrs. A's and Mrs. C's **Medication Records** contain the following information:

Medication Record

Routine	Time
Glyburide 10mg po qd	0800
Tenormin 25 po qd	1100
(patient requests these hours)	
Furosemide 20 mg po bid	1100 - 1700
Cephalothin Sodium IVPB q6h	10- 4-10- 4

PRN Medication
MOM 30 cc prn constipation
Restoril 30 mg po HS may repeat x1

Mrs. A Allergies: None

Medication Record

Routine	Time
Minipress 1 mg po qd	0900
Multivitamin tab i po qd	0900

PRN Medication
MOM 30 cc prn constipation

Mrs. C Allergies: None

Interactive activity: With a partner, **use the case study and the flow charts** to:

1. Identify the pertinent patient information made known to you in the report	2. Identify the pertinent information you gathered from the flow charts	3. Review the data in columns 1 & 2 and identify information that needs follow-up
Mrs. A: • • •	**Mrs. A:** • •	**Mrs. A:** • •
Mrs. C: • • •	**Mrs. C:** •	**Mrs. C:** • • •

It is 0800, **prioritize** your plan of care for both patients for the next 3 hours:

Time	Plan of Nursing Care

➤ You return from lunch at 1200 and Mrs. A is asking for her antihypertensive medication. You know you gave the medication, but she insists that you did not give her the medication. As you investigate, the nursing assistant tells you that Mrs. C is very lethargic and unresponsive. You suddenly realize that you gave Mrs. A's 1100 medications to Mrs. C.

1. Identify the nursing interventions that you would plan to implement immediately	2. Make a nurse's note entry as to how you might document this incident.

For each of the following **nursing interventions**, write an **expected patient outcome**:

1. Prepare for a code ⟹
2. Insert saline lock ⟹

CLINICAL SITUATION - # 10

Intershift taped report at 11:00 PM:

"Mrs. J, 88 years old, was admitted this evening from a nursing home after the family found her lethargic and confused. Her admitting vital signs were T. 101° F - P. 92, irregular - R. 28, short and shallow - B/P 110/70. Her physician was called for admitting orders; he will come in tomorrow morning to see her. She was given Tylenol at 8:30 PM and her current temp. is 100.6° F; she is still slightly confused. The family states that she had cataract surgery 1 week ago as an outpatient. She has an IV going. The patient in the next bed is concerned about Mrs. J's moaning."

Mrs. J's current **flow charts** contain the following information:

Nursing Care Kardex

VS q4h   Diet: DAT

LBM: On admission
IV: 0.9% NS at 75 cc/hr
#24 angio cath RFA

Lab: CBC, Chem panel, UA

PRN Medication:
Tylenol 325 mg tabs ii q4h prn temp > 101° F

Nurse's Notes from Skilled Nursing Facility

Documentation of latest nurse's notes:

1600 Turned, incontinent of urine, strong urine odor, incontinent pad applied. — A. Cann LVN
1700 Family in to visit. Upset, called physician. — A. Cann LVN
1830 Transferred to hospital per order. Recent UA culture reports show + MRSA. Unable to contact physician, copy of report included with transfer. — T. Gage RN

Interactive activity: With a partner, **use the case study and the flow charts** to:

1. Identify the pertinent patient information made known to you in the report	2. Identify the pertinent information you gathered from the flow charts	3. Review the data in columns 1 & 2 and identify information that needs follow-up
•	•	•
•	•	•
•	•	•
•	•	•
•		
•		

It is 11:30 PM, **prioritize** your plan of care for the next hour:

Time	Plan of Nursing Care

➤ Mrs. J is moved to a private room with isolation set up. She slept 1 to 2 hours at a time during the night and remains confused. She has developed a productive cough and is expectorating a small amount of thick creamy yellow-colored phlegm. Her morning vital signs are T. 100.8° F - P. 110 - R. 32 - B/P 114/82. At 6:30 AM the physician visits and leaves the following orders:

Vancomycin 500 mg q6h IVPB
Insert indwelling urinary catheter
Bed rest
Chest x-ray/ECG
Oxygen 2 L/min/NP, pulse oximeter q4h
I & O, enc. fluid intake

1. Identify the nursing interventions that you would plan to implement immediately	2. Identify the instructions you would give to staff and family in caring for Mrs. J

For the following **nursing intervention**, write an **expected patient outcome**:

1. Encourage fluid intake ➡

CLINICAL SITUATION - # 11

Intershift taped report at 11:00 PM:

"The patient is 27 years old and was admitted this evening. He has been diagnosed with viral hepatitis. He is very jaundiced and his urine is very dark yellow. Intake for the shift was 100 cc and output 300 cc. He does not want to eat. He says he has not had an appetite for several days. The IV was started at 5:00 PM and is on time. His 8:00 PM vital signs are T. 37.5° C - P. - 88 - R. 24 - B/P 130/70. He is currently complaining of itching and nausea. The lab reports just arrived and I put them in the patient's chart for the physician to see in the morning."

The patient's current **flow charts** contain the following information:

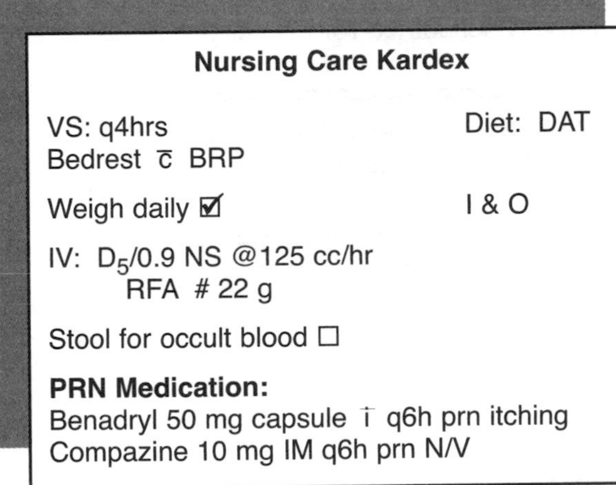

Nursing Care Kardex

VS: q4hrs Diet: DAT
Bedrest c̄ BRP

Weigh daily ☑ I & O

IV: D_5/0.9 NS @125 cc/hr
RFA # 22 g

Stool for occult blood ☐

PRN Medication:
Benadryl 50 mg capsule ī q6h prn itching
Compazine 10 mg IM q6h prn N/V

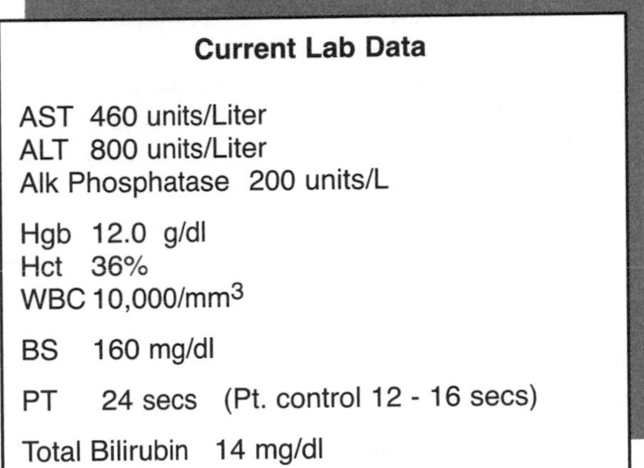

Current Lab Data

AST 460 units/Liter
ALT 800 units/Liter
Alk Phosphatase 200 units/L

Hgb 12.0 g/dl
Hct 36%
WBC 10,000/mm^3

BS 160 mg/dl

PT 24 secs (Pt. control 12 - 16 secs)

Total Bilirubin 14 mg/dl

Interactive activity: With a partner, **use the case study and the flow charts** to:

1. Identify the pertinent patient information made known to you in the report	**2. Identify the pertinent information you gathered from the flow charts**	**3. Review the data in columns 1 & 2 and identify information that needs follow-up**
•	•	•
•		
•	•	•
•	•	•
•	•	•
•	•	•
•	•	•

It is 11:30 p.m., prioritize your plan of care for the next hour:

Time	Plan of Nursing Care

➤ The patient is diagnosed with hepatitis A and is tentatively scheduled for discharge in 2 days

1. Identify the dicharge information that you would include in teaching the patient and his family how best to recover from Hepatitis A.

Diet: **Fluids:** **Nausea/Vomiting:** **Preventing transmission:**	**Activity:** **Skin care:** **Sexual concerns:** **Alcohol intake:** **Follow-up care:**

For the following **nursing intervention**, write the **expected patient outcome**:

1. Patient education ⟹

CLINICAL SITUATION - # 12

Intershift taped report at 7:00 AM:

"Mr. T, 67 years old, has prostate cancer with metastasis to the bone. I have medicated him around the clock for pain, the last dose given at 5:00 AM. He is lethargic but responds when spoken to. He needs frequent mouth care. His urine is amber. The 6:00 AM vital signs are stable at T. 99° F - P. 76 - R. 18 - B/P 126/74. Intake is 100 cc, output is 150 cc. His wife spent the night in the room and is making arrangements for hospice care."

Mr. T's current **flow charts** contain the following information:

Nursing Care Kardex

VS: q4hrs Diet: Soft
Bedrest

Saline lock ☑ I & O
RFA # 22 g

Urinary catheter ☑

PRN Medication:
Meperidine 100 mg q3h IVP prn pain

Allergies: MS

Pt: Mr. T No code

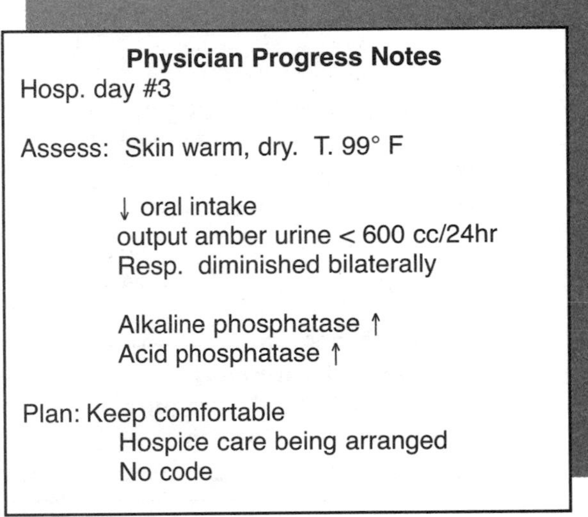

Physician Progress Notes
Hosp. day #3

Assess: Skin warm, dry. T. 99° F

↓ oral intake
output amber urine < 600 cc/24hr
Resp. diminished bilaterally

Alkaline phosphatase ↑
Acid phosphatase ↑

Plan: Keep comfortable
Hospice care being arranged
No code

Interactive activity: With a partner, **use the case study and the flow charts** to:

1. Identify the pertinent patient information made known to you in the report	**2. Identify the pertinent information you gathered from the flow charts**	**3. Review the data in columns 1 & 2 and identify information that needs follow-up**
•	•	•
•	•	•
•	•	•
•	•	•
•	•	
•	•	
•	•	

It is 7:30 AM, **prioritize** your plan of care for the next hour:

Time	**Plan of Nursing Care**

➤ 2:00 PM Mrs. T calls to inform you that Mr. T is in a lot of pain and she is very upset and tells you that the pain shots do not seem to be giving him any comfort. You call the physician and suggest an order for something stronger. The physician orders morphine sulfate 15 mg IVP q3h prn pain. You administer the first dose at 2:15 PM. At 2:25 PM Mrs. T calls you into the room and tells you that her husband is not breathing.

On assessment, you note that Mr. T has stopped breathing and there is no pulse.

1. Identify the nursing interventions that require immediate follow-up	**2. Identify and discuss the ethical issue presented in this situation**

For the following **nursing intervention**, write the **expected patient outcome**:

1. Notify physician of patient's ↑ pain. ⟹

CLINICAL SITUATION - # 13

Intershift taped report at 7:00 AM:

"Mrs. S, 58 years old, is 1 day post op right radical mastectomy. Her dressing is clean and dry. She has a Hemovac that drained 50 cc. Her vital signs at 6:00 AM are T. 99.6° F - P. 88 - R. 24 - B/P 150/90. She is using the PCA and a new liter was hung at 6:00 AM. Her right arm is elevated on a pillow; there is some swelling and she is complaining of some numbness."

Mrs. S's current **flow charts** contain the following information:

Nursing Care Kardex

VS: q4h — Diet: Clear liquid
Up in chair — I & O

IV: Lactated Ringers @ 125 cc/hr
LFA # 18 g — Hemovac ☑

Hgb & Hct this AM ☑

Routine Medications:
Atenolol 50 mg po bid

PRN Medications:
PCA with MS at 1 mg/6 min/pt. demand

History and Physical

The patient is a 58-year-old female, widow. She lives alone. Does not smoke, drinks socially. Has mild hypertension 154/96.
Meds: Atenolol 50 mg po bid
Both parents deceased: mother died of breast cancer, father died of heart disease

Patient has two married daughters and one son

She found a hard lump in the right breast 3 weeks ago. A biopsy was done → Stage II
CEA 5 ng/ml

Plan: Right radical mastectomy
Chemotherapy to follow

Interactive activity: With a partner, **use the case study and the flow charts** to:

1. Identify the pertinent patient information made known to you in the report	2. Identify the pertinent information you gathered from the flow charts	3. Review the data in columns 1 & 2 and identify information that needs follow-up
•	•	•
•	•	•
•	•	•
•	•	•
•	•	•
•	•	•
	•	•
	•	•
	•	

It is 7:30 AM, **prioritize** your plan of care for the next hour:

Time	Plan of Nursing Care

➤ 8:00 AM: You assess the following on Mrs. S: Alert and oriented. VS: T. 99° F - P. 94 – R. 28 - B/P 160/100. Lung sounds with fine rales in the lower bases. Surgical dressing is clean and dry. Hemovac is compressed with 10 cc reddish drainage. Right arm is elevated on a pillow. Finger puffy, c/o of a "numbness sensation." State on a 1-10 pain scale, the pain is at 2. Abdominal sounds present x4. Anti-embolic hose on. Lactated Ringer's infusing, site without redness or swelling, 500 cc left

1. Identify the nursing interventions that require immediate follow-up	2. Identify and discuss the postop educational needs of the patient
	•
	•
	•
	•
	•
	•
	•

For the following **nursing intervention**, write the **expected patient outcome**:

1. Encourage to participate in self-care activities ⟹

CLINICAL SITUATION - # 14

Intershift taped report at 7:00 AM:

"Mr. S has left-sided heart failure. He had a restless night with some dyspnea and a dry non-productive cough most of the night. Crackles are heard in both lungs. He has 3+ pitting edema in both legs and sacrum. His 6:00 AM vital signs are T. 97.6° F - P. 110 irregular - R. 34 -B/P 150/100. His IV site looks slightly puffy, but there is a good blood return. He just started to complain of nausea. His serum K^+ this morning is 3.0 mEq. It might be low because he is retaining fluid. His physician always comes in early so I posted the results in front of the patient's chart."

Mr. S's current **flow charts** contain the following information:

Nursing Care Kardex

VS: q4h — Diet: 2 g NA^+
↑ HOB — I & O
Bedrest with BRP
Weigh qd ☑
LBM (2 days ago)

IV: D_5/0.45 NS $\bar{c}$ 20 mEq KCl — q12h
L hand # 20 g

LAB:
Digoxin level ☑
K^+, NA^+, BUN, Creatinine, AST ☑

DX: CHF — Age: 72

Medication Record

Routine	Time
Digoxin 0.25 mg po qd	0900
Furosemide 40 mg IVP qd	0900 - 1700
K-Dur 10 mEq po BID	0900 - 1700
Capoten 6.25 mg po TID	0900 -1700 - 2200
Colace 100 mg po qd	0900
PRN	
NTG SL gr 1/150 prn chest pain	

Interactive activity: With a partner, **use the case study and the flow charts** to:

1. Identify the pertinent patient information made known to you in the report	2. Identify the pertinent information you gathered from the flow charts	3. Review the data in columns 1 & 2 and identify information that needs follow-up
•	•	•
•	•	•
•	•	•
•	•	•
•	•	•
•	•	•
•	•	•
•	•	•

It is 7:30 AM, **prioritize** your plan of care for the next hour:

Time	Plan of Nursing Care

➤ **9:00 AM** The physician has not come in to see Mr. S. Mr. S is alert but experiencing increasing SOB, cough, and nausea and complaining of blurred vision. His pulse oximetry result is 88%. P. 116 irregular - R. 34, short and shallow - B/P 152/100. Skin cool, color with slight cyanosis. Aside from the K^+ of 3.0 mEq, Mr. S's Na^+ is 135+ mEq, and his digoxin level is 2.4 ng/ml. You call the physician and learn that he is in surgery and will call you back within 30 minutes.

1. Identify the nursing interventions that require immediate follow-up	2. Write a nurse's note to describe the 9:00 AM situation and the follow-up interventions

For the following **nursing intervention**, write the **expected patient outcome**:

1. Lasix 40 mg IVP ⟹

CLINICAL SITUATION - # 15

Intershift taped report at 7:00 AM:

"Mrs. LV, 74 years old, is 4 days post-op left hip fracture. She had a constavac that was removed yesterday. Surgical dressing is clean and dry. Pedal pulse on the left foot is present and the circulation, movement, and sensation are WNL. Lung sounds with fine crackles at the lower bases in both lungs. You need to encourage her to deep breaths and use the incentive spirometer. Her 6:00 AM vital signs are T. 99.8° F - P. 80 - R. 18 - B/P 130/82. She does not want to move, it seems like she is scared. I have medicated her two times during the night."

Mrs. LV's current **flow charts** contain the following information:

Nursing Care Kardex

VS: qs — Diet: Soft
HOH — I & O
Ambulate with PT

LBM (2 days ago)

IV: Saline lock LFA #22g angio cath
Inserted day of surgery

Routine Medications:

Digoxin 0.125 mg po qd	9
Furosemide 10 mg po qd	9
$FeSO_4$ 300 mg po tid c̄ meals	8-12-5

PRN:
Vicodin tab i̅ q4h prn pain

Medical History

Elderly female brought into the ED after falling at home. A fracture of the left hip was diagnosed. She was taken to surgery and an ORIF was performed.
Hgb 9.4 mg/dl, Hct 28% on admission.

She lives alone, has one son and her husband died 2 years ago from a cardiac condition.

Patient has a history of atrial fibrillation.

Interactive activity: With a partner, **use the case study and the flow charts** to:

1. Identify the pertinent patient information made known to you in the report	2. Identify the pertinent information you gathered from the flow charts	3. Review the data in columns 1 & 2 and identify information that needs follow-up
•	•	•
•	•	•
•	•	•
•	•	•
•	•	•
•	•	•
•	•	
•	•	

It is 7:30 AM, prioritize your plan of care for the next hour:

Time	Plan of Nursing Care

➤ **You review the nurse's notes from the night shift and note the following:**

12:00 PM Alert, moaning, states leg hurts. Circulation, movement, and sensation of left leg WNL. Dressing clean and dry. Repositioned. Vicodin tab ī given for pain.
2:00 AM Awake, states pain in leg, does not want to be touched. Left pedal pulse palpable. Repositioned.
4:00 AM Sleeping
6:00 AM c/o leg pain. Medicated with Vicodin tab ī.

You enter the following assessment in the nurse's notes:

7:30 AM Awake, alert, states "did not have a good night." c/o leg pain. Left leg with pedal pulse, warm, cap. refill >2 sec. Leg elevated on pillow. Dressing clean and dry. Right leg with weak pedal pulse, swelling and redness noted at calf and thigh. Tender to touch. Lung sounds with fine crackles, encouraged to take deep breaths. Bowel sounds present x4, c/o constipation.

1. Identify the nursing interventions that require immediate follow-up	2. Identify the instructions that you will give the nursing assistants at this time

For the following **nursing intervention**, write the **expected patient outcome**:

1. Elevation of right leg ⟹

CLINICAL SITUATION - # 16

Intershift taped report at 3:00 PM:

"Mrs. L was admitted with signs and symptoms of having developed a pulmonary embolism. She just had a baby 2 weeks ago. She has a heparin drip. The infusion pump is set at 20 cc/hr. You have 100 cc left. She slept well. Respirations are unlabored at 22. The right lower lung has diminished breath sounds. She will be started on coumadin today. She is anxious to go home and be with her baby."

Mrs. L's current **flow charts** contain the following information:

Nursing Care Kardex

VS: q4h Diet: Regular

Bedrest with BRP I & O
O_2 @ 3 L/min/NC prn SOB

IV: 500 cc D_5W $\bar{c}$ 20,000 U Heparin
LFA # 22 g angio cath
Infuse at 1000 U/hr

LAB:
Daily PTT ☑ PT in AM

Routine Medications:
Coumadin 5 mg po today at 0900
Coumadin 2.5 mg po today at 1700

Coagulation Record

Date	PTT	Control	Heparin dose
1st day	50 sec	25 sec	900 U/hr
2nd day	60 sec	25 sec	1000 U/hr
3rd day	90 sec	30 sec	1100 U/hr
Current	75 sec	30 sec	1000 U/hr

Interactive activity: With a partner, **use the case study and the flow charts** to:

1. Identify the pertinent patient information made known to you in the report	2. Identify the pertinent information you gathered from the flow charts	3. Review the data in columns 1 & 2 and identify information that needs follow-up
• • • • •	• • • • • • • • •	• • • • • •

It is 3:30 PM, **prioritize** your plan of care for the next hour:

Time	Plan of Nursing Care

➤ **6:30 PM** The nursing assistant informs you that the IV pump is beeping. You go into assess the pump and you notice that the heparin bag empty. You look at the infusion pump and it is set at 35 cc/hr.

1. Identify the nursing interventions that require immediate follow-up	2. Document your findings as you would enter them in the nursing notes

For the following **nursing intervention**, write the **expected patient outcome**:

1. Monitor for signs and symptoms of bleeding ⟹

CLINICAL SITUATION - # 17

Intershift taped report at 3:00 PM:

"Ms. P, 23 years old, had an emergency appendectomy yesterday. She has Down syndrome. She has gotten up to the chair twice today. Surgical dressing is clean, dry, and intact. Bowel sounds are hypoactive. Her IV is infusing well; you have 200 cc left. Oral intake is 100 cc and output is the 400 cc. I have medicated her at noon for pain. Her noon vital signs are T. 100° F - P. 80 - R. 20 - B/P 110/78."

Ms. P's current **flow charts** contain the following information:

Nursing Care Kardex

VS: q4h　　Diet: Clear liquid

Ambulate c̄ assistance　　I & O

IV: IL D_5/0.9 NS @ 125 cc/hr
LFA # 22 g angio cath

Routine Medications:
Cefoxitin 2 g IVPB q6h 10 - 4 - 10 - 4

PRN Medications:
Morphine Sulfate 8 mg IV q4h prn pain
Droperidol 1.25 mg IV q4h prn N/V

Intake and Output Record

7 – 3 shift:

Intake		Output		
Oral:	100	Void:	8:00 AM	50
			9:00	50
			11:00	75
			12:00	50
			1:00 PM	75
IV:	900		2:00	100
IVPB:	50			
		Emesis	12:00 PM	100
Total:	1050		Total:	500

Interactive activity: With a partner, **use the case study and the flow charts** to:

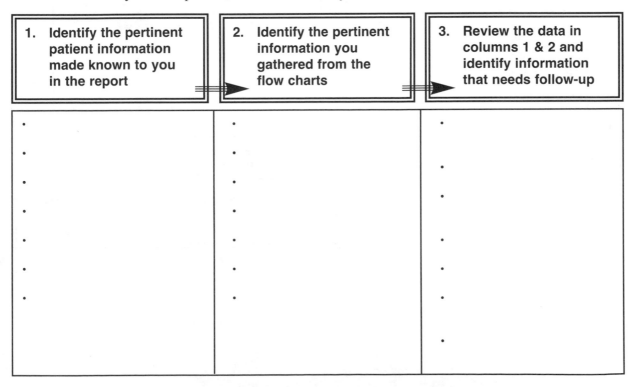

1. Identify the pertinent patient information made known to you in the report	**2. Identify the pertinent information you gathered from the flow charts**	**3. Review the data in columns 1 & 2 and identify information that needs follow-up**
•	•	•
•	•	•
•	•	•
•	•	•
•	•	•
•	•	•
•	•	•
		•

It is 3:30 PM, **prioritize** your plan of care for the next hour:

Time	Plan of Nursing Care

➤ **8:00 PM** Ms. P's mother and family are at the bedside. They tell you that Ms. P is increasingly restless and is pulling at her surgical dressing. You note the following entries in the nursing notes:

Has voided a total of 100 cc since 4:00 PM. Emesis 100 cc greenish fluid at 6:00 PM, refused dinner. Morphine sulfate 8 mg and droperidol 1.25 mg given IV at 6:00 PM.

1. Identify the nursing interventions that require immediate follow-up	2. Identify a rationale for each nursing intervention that you plan to implement

For the following **nursing intervention**, write the **expected patient outcome**:

1. Ambulate patient ⟹

CLINICAL SITUATION - # 18

Intershift taped report at 0700:

"Mr. O has cellulitis of the right leg. He is pretty much self-care and he says he is not used to being in bed so much. He stays in a chair most of the time with his leg elevated. His I & O is fine and his vital signs are stable at T. 37° C - P. 92 - R. 22 - B/P 164/94. He has a dry dressing on the right leg and there is no drainage. His saline lock needs to be changed today and his fingerstick blood sugar was 110 this morning."

Mr. O's current **flow charts** contain the following information:

Nursing Care Kardex

VS: q4h Diet: 2000 cal ADA
BRP
4x4 to right leg - Change qs
LBM 1 day ago I & O
IV: Saline lock
LFA # 22 g angio cath

Heating pad to right leg
Elevate leg on pillow

Fingerstick BS qAM 0600 ☑
C. O 62 yrs. Dx: Cellulits R. Leg
Hx: Angina, Hypertension, DM type 2

Medication Record

Routine:

Glyburide 10 mg po qd		0800	
Verapamil SR 240 mg po	bid	0900	1700
Inderal 20 mg po bid		0900	1700
ASA 81 mg po qd		0900	
Colace 100 mg po qd		0900	

Velosef 2 g IVPB q6h 2400-0600-1200-1800

PRN:
NTG SL gr 1/150 q5min × 3 prn chest pain

Interactive activity: With a partner, **use the case study and the flow charts** to:

1. Identify the pertinent patient information made known to you in the report	2. Identify the pertinent information you gathered from the flow charts	3. Review the data in columns 1 & 2 and identify information that needs follow-up
•	•	•
•	•	•
•	•	•
•	•	•
•	•	•
•	•	•
•	•	

It is 0730, **prioritize** your plan of care for the next hour:

Time	Plan of Nursing Care

➤ **1200:** Mr. O returns to bed after having a BM. You note that he is SOB and his skin is cool and clammy. You assess his vital signs, his radial pulse is 110 and irregular, respirations are 32, and his B/P is 170/100. He tells you that he is feeling pressure on his chest. You assist him into bed and place him in high Fowler's position.

1. Identify your follow-up nursing interventions	2. Identify a rationale for each nursing intervention that you plan to implement

For the following **nursing intervention**, write the **expected patient outcome**:

1. Administration of oxygen ⟹

CLINICAL SITUATION - # 19

Intershift taped report at 7:00 AM:

"Mr. I, 70 years old, is 1 day post-op a TURP. He has a continuous normal saline irrigation. I will hang up a new irrigation bag before I leave. He has had several clots during the shift. His vital signs are T. 37.2° C - P. 90 - R. 22 - B/P 160/93. He is alert and cheerful, and told me that he leads a very active life. I gave him a suppository for c/o bladder spasms at 5 this morning. The IV is also very positional."

Mr. I's current **flow charts** contain the following information:

Nursing Care Rand

VS q4h Diet: Clear liquids
Antiembolic hose on
LBM: On admission
IV: Lactated Ringer's at 75 cc/hr
#20 angio cath RFA

3-way indwelling cath c̄ 30-cc balloon
NS con't irrigation - keep UA free of clots

Routine Medication:
Colace 100 mg po qAM 1000

PRN Medication:
B & O supp. i q6h prn bladder spasms

Intake and Output Record

11-7 shift:

Intake		Output
Oral -		50
1300		
		(NS irrigation 1000)
IV:	300	
Total:	350	300

Interactive activity: With a partner, **use the case study and the flow charts** to:

1. Identify the pertinent patient information made known to you in the report	2. Identify the pertinent information you gathered from the flow charts	3. Review the data in columns 1 & 2 and identify information that needs follow-up
•	•	•
•	•	•
•	•	•
•	•	•
•	•	•
•	•	
	•	

It is 7:30 AM, **prioritize** your plan of care for the next hour:

Time	Plan of Nursing Care

➤ **8:00 AM:** Mr. I is complaining of increased pain. He is grimacing, is diaphoretic and tells you he has an urge to urinate. You note that the irrigation bag is empty and there are 50 cc of burgundy-colored urine in the urinary collection bag. There is urine leaking around the catheter.

1. **Identify the nursing interventions that you would plan to implement immediately**	2. **Identify the follow-up nursing interventions for the rest of the shift**

For the following **nursing interventions**, write **expected patient outcomes**:

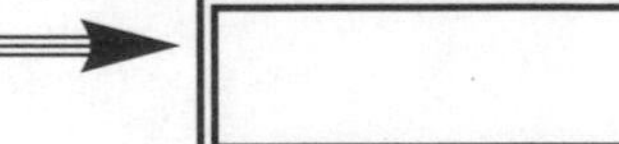

1. Bladder irrigation ⟹
2. Enc. fluid intake ⟹

CLINICAL SITUATION - # 20

Intershift taped report at 7:00 AM:

"Mrs. F, 46 years old, had a TAH-BSO yesterday. She had soft bowel sounds this morning. The abdominal dressing is clean and dry. Her IV is infusing well and she has an epidural infusion with fentanyl infusing through a pump. She has not had any break through pain. The epidural dressing is intact and the catheter is fine. She has been mostly on bed rest, but she is to get up to a chair this morning. The 6:00 AM vital signs are T. 37.5° C - P. 78 - R. 18 - B/P 130/80. Her output was 500 cc."

Mrs. F's current **flow charts** contain the following information:

Nursing Care Rand

VS: q4h Diet: Clear liquids
Up in chair with assistance
Incentive spirometer q1h ×10 WA
LBM: Prior to admission

Urinary catheter ☑

IV: D_5/0.45 NS q8h

Routine Medication:
Fentanyl 6 cc/hr in NS via epidural catheter ordered by anesthesiologist

Intake and Output Record

Night shift:

Intake		Output	
Oral (Sips of H_2O)	50	Void	
		UA cath	500
IV:	1000		
IV (Fentanyl)	48		

Interactive activity: With a partner, **use the case study and the flow charts** to:

1. Identify the pertinent patient information made known to you in the report	2. Identify the pertinent information you gathered from the flow charts	3. Review the data in columns 1 & 2 and identify information that needs follow-up
•	•	•
•	•	•
•	•	•
•	•	•
•	•	•
•		
•		

It is 7:30 AM, **prioritize** your plan of care for the next hour:

Time	Plan of Nursing Care

➤ **At 8:30 AM** Mrs. F gets up with assistance to sit in a chair. As she walks slowly to the chair, she steps on some of the tubings. The nursing assistant tells you that the infusion pump is beeping. You go into assess and note that the epidural infusion pump it beeping and the patient's epidural dressing is pulled from the patient's back. The epidural catheter seems to be pulled out.

1. Identify the nursing interventions that you would plan to implement immediately	2. Document your findings as you would enter them in the nursing notes

For the following **nursing intervention**, write an **expected patient outcome**:

1. Cover epidural site with 4 × 4 ⟹

SECTION FOUR

Management and Leadership

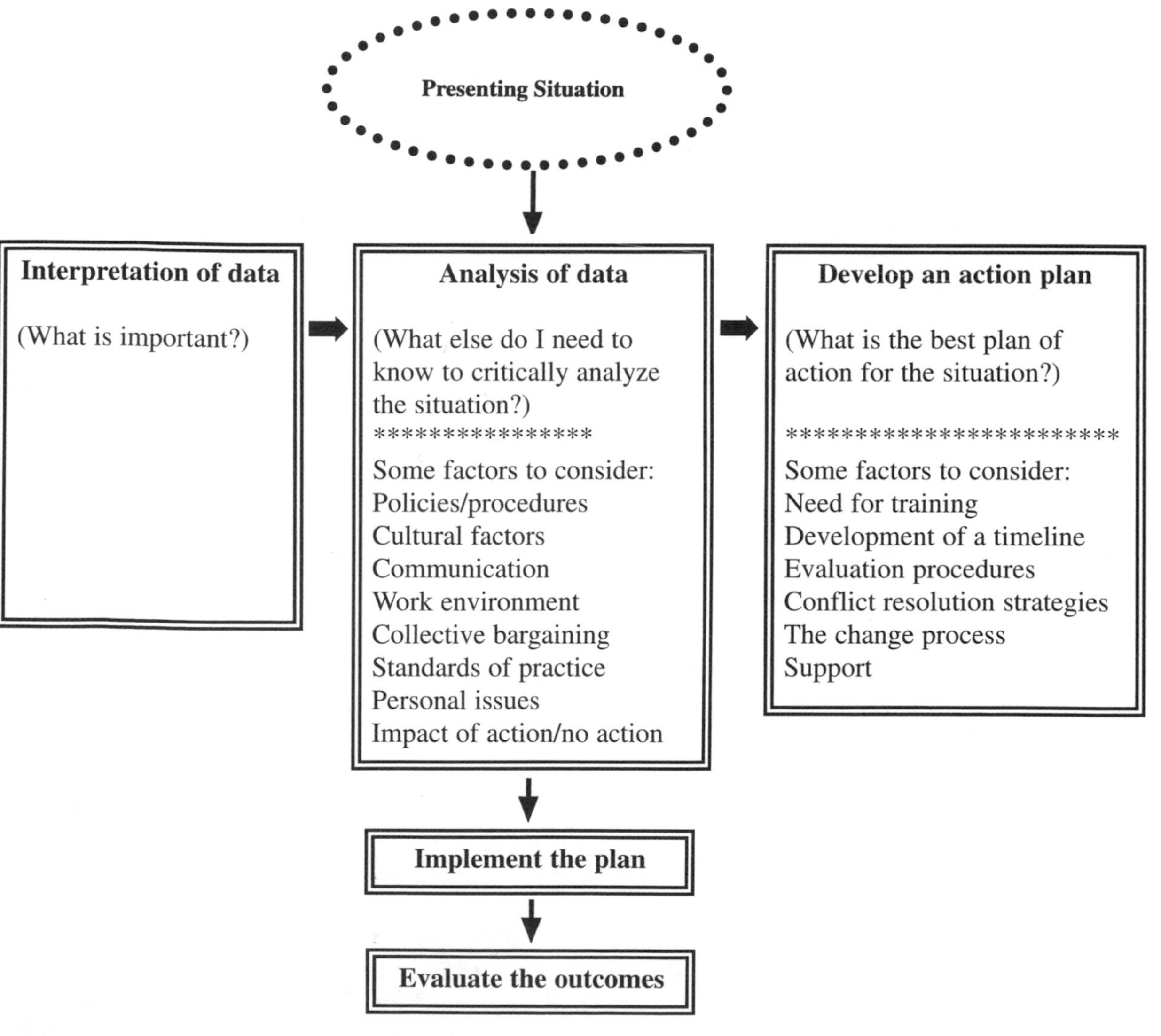

Presenting Situation
Interpretation of data
(What is important?)
Analysis of data
(What else do I need to know to critically analyze the situation?)
****
Some factors to consider:
Policies/procedures
Cultural factors
Communication
Work environment
Collective bargaining
Standards of practice
Personal issues
Impact of action/no action
Develop an action plan
(What is the best plan of action for the situation?)
****
Some factors to consider:
Need for training
Development of a timeline
Evaluation procedures
Conflict resolution strategies
The change process
Support
Implement the plan
Evaluate the outcomes

MANAGEMENT AND LEADERSHIP

CLINICAL SITUATION - # 1

The supervisor of a medical unit has recently hired several new RNs just out of nursing school. Two of the new RNs have started on the day shift. As an RN with 7 years experience, you have been assigned to orient and precept one of the new RNs. The new RN will work with you for 3 months.

Information about the experienced RN: You have worked mainly on the medical unit and are considered an expert. You are always on time. You are organized and can be counted on "to get the job done." You are frequently given all of the new employees to orient. You have never complained and you like working with nurses, but you are getting pretty tired of having to be the one that is assigned to orient the new employees all the time.

Information about the new RN: He is in his twenties, quiet but friendly. He works steadily, has a good knowledge base, but has difficulty asking questions. He has managed the care of three patients in school. He was late the first day on the unit and tells the nurse that he "is more of a night person."

1. Identify the strong and weak characteristics demonstrated in the RNs.

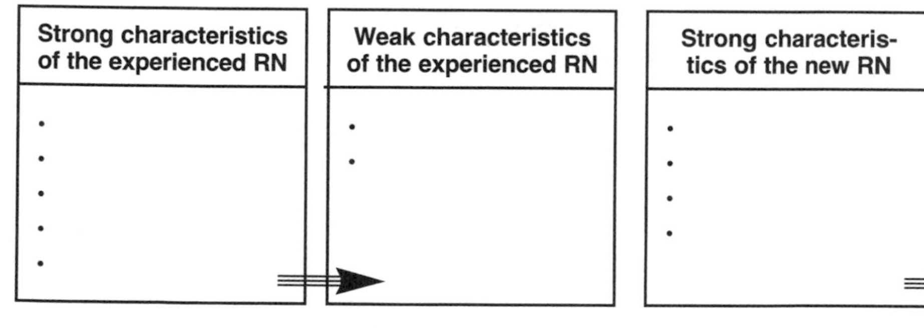

Strong characteristics of the experienced RN
•
•
•
•
•
Weak characteristics of the experienced RN
•
•

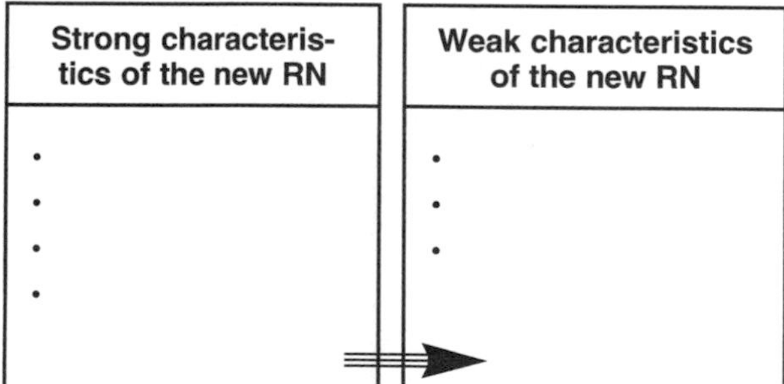

Strong characteristics of the new RN
•
•
•
•
Weak characteristics of the new RN
•
•
•

2. Prioritize the one major issue that may cause conflict initially.

1. ______________________________

____

____

As the experienced RN, how would you handle this major issue?

____

____

Before implementing the plan, what other issues should be considered?

____

____

Clinical situation continued:

As the experienced nurse, you develop the following goals to help guide the progress of the new RN. You discuss these goals with the new RN.

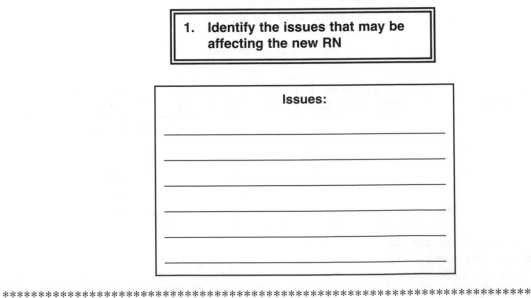

Goals for the first week:

-
-
-
-

Goals for the second week:

-
-
-
-
-
-

At the end of the 2 weeks, the new RN has not been able to achieve the set goals. The experienced RN sets up a time to meet with the new RN. During the meeting, the new RN is visibly upset.

1. Identify the issues that may be affecting the new RN

Issues:

____

____

____

____

____

____

****

With a partner, role play the part of the experienced nurse and the new RN.

As the experienced RN, how would you handle this situation?

____

____

____

____

____

____

____

As the new RN, how would you like this situation handled?

____

____

____

____

____

____

____

MANAGEMENT AND LEADERSHIP

CLINICAL SITUATION - # 3

An RN transferred to the medical unit after working 5 years in the ICU. It has taken some time—3 months to be exact—to organize and manage the care of 5 to 6 patients assigned to her on the day shift. The majority of the patients are high acuity and have multiple problems. Most of the staff has been very supportive, always checking to see if they can help. However, the RN has observed one nursing assistant who rarely helps out the other staff members. On several occasions the RN has believed that some interventions that the the nursing assistant has done have been performed incorrectly.

Information about the RN: The RN is used to working independently. She would rather do the procedure or provide the care herself to ensure that it is done correctly. This has been a difficult transition for her since she has to rely on ancillary help to complete her work. Although the RN can delegate many tasks, she finds herself avoiding this nursing assistant and mostly doing the tasks herself. She stays late everyday to complete the charting on the patients.

Information about the nursing assistant: The nursing assistant has been on this unit for 1 year. She feels pretty comfortable with her skills and has even shown other nursing assistants how to take short cuts. She enjoys working by herself and takes pride in not asking anyone for help. She does not like being told how to do something that she already knows how to do. She is frustrated with the RN since the RN seems to be running around in circles. As far as she is concerned, she will do her job, and, unless asked, she will not do anything extra.

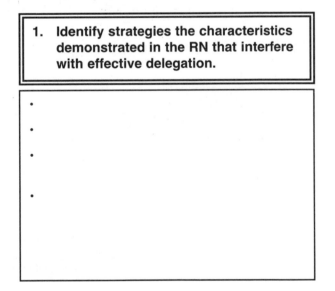

1. Identify strategies the characteristics demonstrated in the RN that interfere with effective delegation.

-
-
-
-

In managing this situation, what can the RN do to work with the problem and create a more conducive working environment with the nursing assistant?

____

____

Clinical situation #3 continued:

The following day the nursing assistant is assigned to work with the RN. There are numerous tasks that need to be done on the patients. The nurse has the following tasks that need to be done for the assigned patients: vital signs, 3 bedbaths, assessments, saline lock irrigations, emptying urinary collection bags on 2 patients, emptying a J-P device, W-D dressing change, passing narcotic medications, applying restraints, monitoring IV fluids, NG tube bolus feeding, oral suctioning, deep suctioning, pulse oximetry, starting oxygen per nasal cannula.

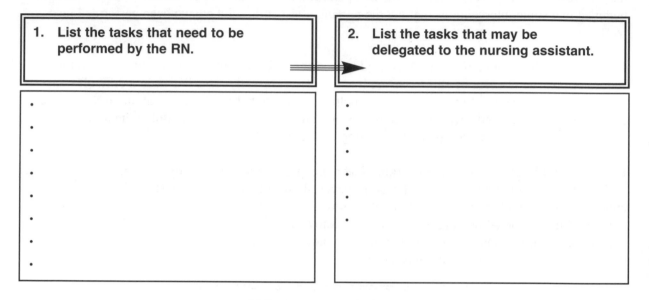

1. List the tasks that need to be performed by the RN.	2. List the tasks that may be delegated to the nursing assistant.
•	•
•	•
•	•
•	•
•	•
•	•
•	
•	

List the criteria that should be considered before delegating a task to another person.

____

____

****

After the RN has taken her own noon vital signs, the nursing assistant approaches her and asks her why she did not let her take the noon vitals on the patients.

With a partner, role play the part of the RN and the nursing assistant.

As the RN, how would you problem-solve this situation?	As the nursing assistant, what would you like to come out of this situation?
______________________________	______________________________
______________________________	______________________________
______________________________	______________________________
______________________________	______________________________
______________________________	______________________________
______________________________	______________________________
______________________________	______________________________

MANAGEMENT AND LEADERSHIP

CLINICAL SITUATION - # 4

Two RNs have worked the day shift together on the oncology unit for several years. Both are expert nurses and through the years they have become close personal friends. RN Nurse A has accepted the position of charge nurse of the oncology unit, and RN Nurse B continues as a staff nurse. For the last 6 months, the charge nurse has been concerned about numerous discrepancies in the narcotics count. Lately, an increasing number of patients have been complaining that they are not obtaining pain relief after being medicated. After a careful investigation by the administrative staff, it was noted that all of the narcotic count discrepancies occurred on the day shift. RN Nurse A is the only person informed of the current findings. A follow-up investigation will be conducted.

Information about the RN Nurse A: The RN is married and has two children. She is frequently involved with the school activities of the children. She loves the staff and enjoys her work but is still learning the duties of a manager. She has a difficult time supervising and evaluating staff and seems to avoid handling any conflict situations. She has noticed that RN Nurse B has been irritable but has assumed that her marital separation is contributing to her behavior. After assessing the behaviors of RN Nurse B, she is wondering whether her friend may be involved.

Information about the RN Nurse B: The RN has two children in school and has recently separated from her husband. She has been unable to be active in her children's school activities because of the added demands brought on by the separation. She has been suffering from migraine headaches but cannot afford to miss any work since the couple had just purchased a new home before the separation. She has asked RN Nurse A to assign her to extra shifts or overtime whenever possible.

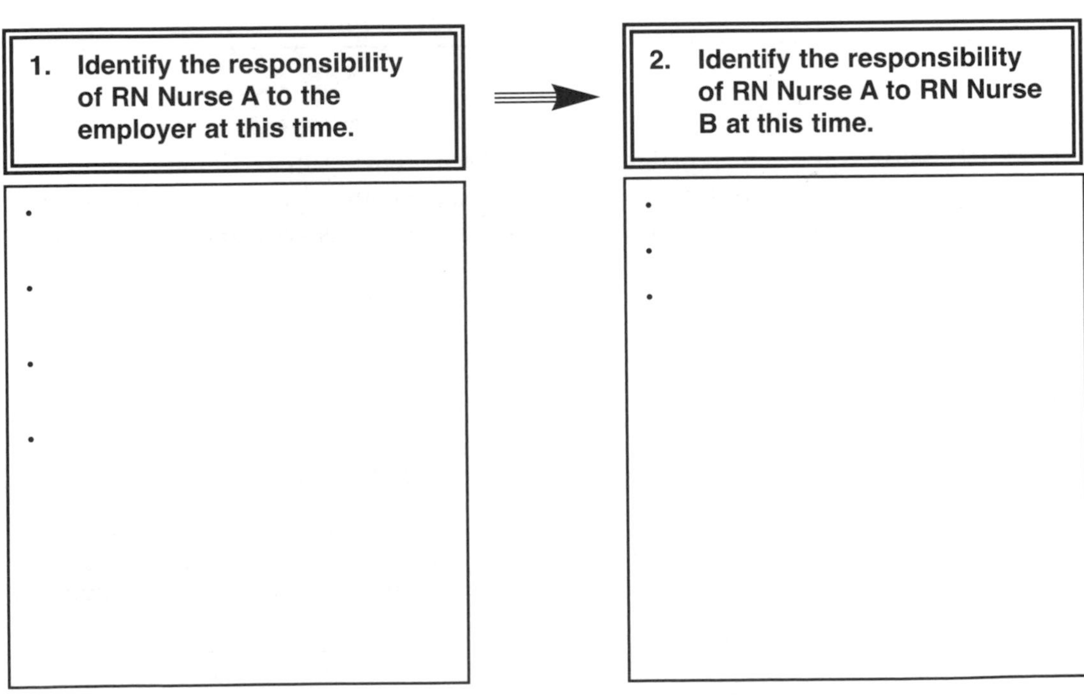
1. Identify the responsibility of RN Nurse A to the employer at this time.
2. Identify the responsibility of RN Nurse A to RN Nurse B at this time.

RN Nurse A feels that she is not being honest with the staff by not sharing the preliminary findings of the investigation. Identify issues that should be considered in this situation.

____

____

Clinical situation #4 continued:

For 3 weeks the narcotic count has been correct. Today, RN Nurse B is assigned to a terminally ill patient. She is preparing to administer pain medication to a patient and takes a syringe labeled morphine sulfate 10 mg from the narcotic drawer. She administers the morphine sulfate IV to the patient. 30 minutes later the patient is moaning with pain and the family is very upset seeing him in such pain. The physician is called and an order for a stat dose of morphine sulfate 5 mg IV is given. RN Nurse A administers the drug to the patient since RN Nurse B is at lunch. The patient is calm for the next 2 hours. RN Nurse A informs RN Nurse B about the additional dose of pain medication given to the patient. At the end of the shift, there is a discrepancy with the morphine sulfate and the narcotic count.

1. Identify the responsibility of RN Nurse A to the employer at this time.	→	**2. Identify the responsibility of RN Nurse A to RN Nurse B at this time.**
• • •		• • •

****

The next day, RN Nurse B is again preparing to administer morphine sulfate 10 mg IV to the patient. RN Nurse B emptied the contents of the morphine sulfate into another syringe and put this syringe in her pocket. She then filled the current syringe with saline and took this syringe into the room and gave the saline to the patient.

RN Nurse A noticed that RN Nurse B had a syringe with liquid in her pocket as she was going home. RN Nurse A confronts RN Nurse B. RN Nurse B tells her friend that it is saline, but she refuses to discard it or to give it to RN Nurse A.

With a partner, role play the part of the RN Nurse A and the RN Nurse B.

As RN Nurse A, how would you handle this situation?	**As RN Nurse B, what would you like to come out of this situation?**
______________________________ ______________________________ ______________________________ ______________________________ ______________________________ ______________________________	______________________________ ______________________________ ______________________________ ______________________________ ______________________________ ______________________________

MANAGEMENT AND LEADERSHIP

CLINICAL SITUATION - # 5

The RN works on an endocrine unit in a hospital that uses a team approach to deliver patient care. The team consists of an RN, an LVN, and two nursing assistants. The RN is responsible for the supervision and the delegation of care. A new, highly recommended LVN has recently been hired to work on the unit. During the first week of orientation, the supervising RN noticed that the LVN was friendly but did not check the insulin dosages with anyone before giving the insulin injections to the patients. The RN told the LVN to have all insulin dosages double-checked before giving. The LVN told one of the nursing assistants that the RN did not trust her. Later, the RN again saw the LVN giving an insulin injection to another patient without checking the insulin dose. The RN questioned the LVN and the LVN coldly responded that she forgot since she never had to have her worked checked in her previous job and she would try to remember next time.

Information about the RN: The RN has been working on the endocrine unit for 2 years. She is very conscientious and, since she has diabetes mellitus, she takes a special interest in working with patients who have diabetes. She works closely with her staff and has not had any serious staff problems. She can tell that the LVN has a lot of experience and is willing to work with her. The RN has little patience for what she considers "unsafe practice" behaviors.

Information about the LVN: The LVN has been a nurse for 15 years. She has worked in several hospitals. In her last job, she worked in a skilled facility where she had increased responsibility. She decided to return to the acute care setting since it offered better financial benefits. She feels that she has a lot of experience and knows more than some of the new RNs. She can tell that the staff RN is recently out of school.

1. Identify the strong and weak characteristics demonstrated in each nurse.

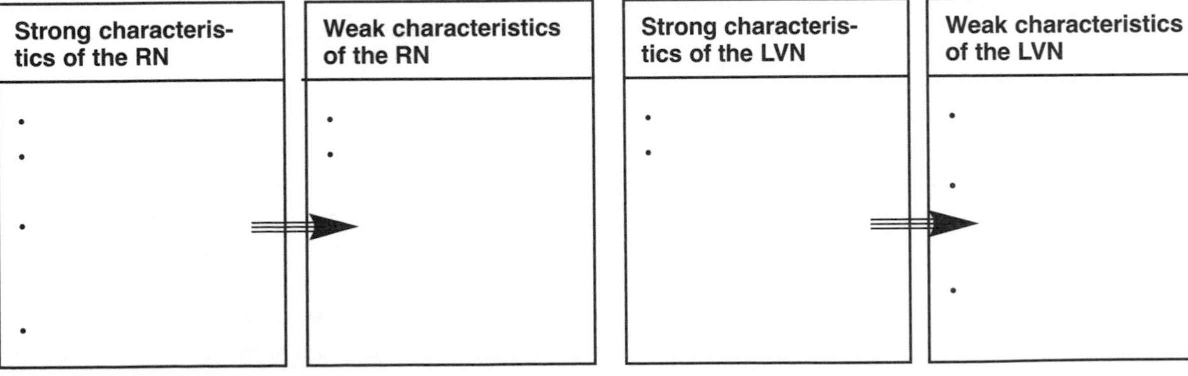

2. Prioritize the major issue that needs to be addressed at this time.

1. ______________________

____

____

As the RN, how would you handle this situation?

____

____

____

____

Clinical situation #5 continued:

For the next 2 weeks, the RN noticed that the LVN had been double-checking the insulin dosages. Today, the unit is very busy and one patient in particular is very upset and requested to speak with the RN. The patient complained of several things but was especially upset because the LVN was going to give him the wrong dose of insulin this morning. The patient explained that he asked the LVN how much insulin she was giving him and that she said 10 U of NPH. The patient insisted that he normally was given 12 U of NPH every morning. The LVN checked and the patient was correct.

The RN discussed the patient's comments with the LVN. The LVN agreed with the patient's comments, telling the RN that it really wasn't a big issue since the dose was a little less than ordered and it could have easily been corrected. The RN decided to set up a meeting with the LVN to discuss the incident further and to present the following anecdotal note:

12/31 0900 Patient X complained that the LVN was going to administer 10 U of NPH insulin to him this morning instead of the usual 12 U he gets every morning. The LVN rechecked the ordered amount and proceeded to administer the correct dose to the patient.

I have told the LVN to double-check all insulin dosages before administering the injection to the patients. The LVN does not realize the seriousness of this behavior.

Discuss, evaluate, and rewrite the anecdotal note.

Anecdotal notes should contain:

-
-
-
-
-
-
-
-

****

The RN meets with the LVN.

With a partner, role play the part of the RN and the LVN.

As RN Nurse A, how would you handle this situation?

____

____

____

____

____

____

____

____

Identify key points to keep in mind when conducting an evaluation meeting with an employee.

-
-
-
-
-

SECTION FIVE

Applying Critical Thinking Skills to Test Questions

Applying Critical Thinking Skills to Test Questions

INSTRUCTIONS: Circle the one best answer for each test question. Write your rationale for selecting the answer. To enhance your learning and test-taking skill, discuss your answer and rationale with a partner. The answer and the rationale can be found on the back of this page.

1. The nurse is demonstrating how to minimize occlusion of a feeding tube after medication administration. Which nursing intervention is most important to include in the demonstration?
   a. Withdraw any residual, give the medication, and flush with 30 ml of water.
   b. Flush the tube before and after giving the medication with 20 ml of water.
   c. Use 30 ml of lukewarm water to flush the tube after giving the medication.
   d. Inject 15 cc of air before and after giving the medication.

   Rationale: ______________________________

2. The client is discharged on phenytoin 100 mg po due at 0800-1600-2400 and an antacid 30 ml prn. For effective drug administration, discharge instructions should include to
   a. administer the phenytoin with a dose of antacid.
   b. skip a dose of the phenytoin if the antacid is taken.
   c. take half the dose of antacid if given with the phenytoin.
   d. avoid taking the antacid at the same time as the phenytoin.

   Rationale: ______________________________

3. The client is receiving TPN through a single-lumen central catheter per infusion pump. Ceftriaxone 1 g in 100 ml 0.9% NaCl is ordered qd IVPB. To safely administer this IVPB, the nurse plans to
   a. hang the IVPB through a Y-port tubing above the infusion pump.
   b. hang the IVPB through a Y-port tubing below the infusion pump.
   c. start a peripheral line for the IVPB.
   d. use a mini-drip tubing for the IVPB.

   Rationale: ______________________________

Applying Critical Thinking Skills to Test Questions

HELPFUL HINTS: Read all test questions carefully. Identify key words in the question that will guide you in answering the question. In these test questions the key words to consider are **"most important," "effective drug administration,"** and **"safely."** Compare your rationale with the one in the test question.

1. The nurse is demonstrating how to minimize occlusion of a feeding tube after medication administration. Which nursing intervention is most important to include in the demonstration?
   a. Withdraw any residual, give the medication, and flush with 30 ml of water.
   (b) Flush the tube before and after giving the medication with 20 ml of water.
   c. Use 30 ml of lukewarm water to flush the tube after giving the medication.
   d. Inject 15 cc of air before and after giving the medication.

   Rationale: **(B) is the answer. It is important to initially check the placement of the NG tube to ensure that the tube and suction are working. Options (a), (c), and (d) do not present the proper technique for administering medications through a feeding tube.**

2. The client is discharged on phenytoin 100 mg po due at 0800-1600-2400 and an antacid 30 ml prn. For effective drug administration, discharge instructions should include to
   a. administer the phenytoin with a dose of antacid.
   b. skip a dose of the phenytoin if the antacid is taken.
   c. take half the dose of antacid if given with the phenytoin.
   (d) avoid taking the antacid at the same time as the phenytoin.

   Rationale: **(D) is the answer. Absorption of phenytoin may be decreased when taken together with an antacid. Options (a) and (c) do not address the effects of an antacid on phenytoin. Drug therapy should not be altered, therefore option (b) is not correct.**

3. The client is receiving TPN through a single-lumen central catheter per infusion pump. Ceftriaxone 1 g in 100 ml 0.9% NaCl is ordered qd IVPB. To safely administer this IVPB, the nurse plans to
   a. hang the IVPB through a Y-port tubing above the infusion pump.
   b. hang the IVPB through a Y-port tubing below the infusion pump.
   (c.) start a peripheral line for the IVPB.
   d. use a mini-drip tubing for the IVPB.

   Rationale: **(C) is the answer. IVPBs cannot be administered in a TPN line. Options (a) and (b) do not safely administer the IVPB because the TPN is used. Option (d) can be used but does not identify how the IVPB will be administered.**

Applying Critical Thinking Skills to Test Questions

INSTRUCTIONS: Circle the one best answer for each test question. Write your rationale for selecting the answer. To enhance your learning and test-taking skill, discuss your answer and rationale with a partner. The answer and the rationale can be found on the back of this page.

1. The nurse learns in report that the serum potassium level of a client is 5.5 mEq/L this morning. The client's doctor is in surgery, so a message is left at the doctor's office. The client is on the following medications at 0800: famotidine 20 mg po and spironolactone 50 mg po. Which action by the nurse is most appropriate?
   a. Hold the morning dose of famotidine until the doctor returns the call.
   b. Hold the morning dose of spironolactone until the doctor returns the call.
   c. Hold all the morning medications until the doctor returns the call.
   d. Give all the morning medications as ordered.

   Rationale: ______________________________

2. The nurse is caring for a client with diabetes mellitus type 2. The following medications are listed on the client's medication record: metformin (Glucophage) 0.5 g po bid and repaglinide (Prandil) 1 mg po with meals. The morning blood glucose fingerstick is 98 mg/dl. Which action by the nurse is most appropriate?
   a. Hold the morning po medications.
   b. Give the metformin, but hold the repaglinide.
   c. Give the repaglinide, but hold the metformin.
   d. Give the po medications as ordered.

   Rationale: ______________________________

3. The client with end-stage renal disease is scheduled for hemodialysis in 2 hours. He has a L AV fistula and needs assistance with feeding. In delegating the care of the client, which nursing order is of priority?
   a. Feed the client first.
   b. Give all morning care before the dialysis.
   c. Take the blood pressure in the right arm.
   d. Feel for a vibration on the left arm.

   Rationale: ______________________________

Applying Critical Thinking Skills to Test Questions

HELPFUL HINTS: : Read all test questions carefully. Identify key words in the question that will guide you in answering the question. In these test questions the **key words** to consider are **"most appropriate"** and **"priority."** Compare your rationale with the one in the test question.

1. The nurse learns in report that the serum potassium level of a client is 5.5 mEq/L this morning. The client's doctor is in surgery, so a message is left at the doctor's office. The client is on the following medications at 0800: famotidine 20 mg po and spironolactone 50 mg po. Which action by the nurse is most appropriate?
   a. Hold the morning dose of famotidine until the doctor returns the call.
   (b.) Hold the morning dose of spironolactone until the doctor returns the call.
   c. Hold all the morning medications until the doctor returns the call.
   d. Give all the morning medications as ordered.

   Rationale: **(B) is the answer. Spironolactone is a potassium-sparing diuretic. Since the morning serum K+ level is high, the drug should be held and until further orders are obtained from the doctor. Option (a) does not affect the potassium level. Options (c) and (d) do not correlate the effects of the specific drugs to the lab work.**

2. The nurse is caring for a client with diabetes mellitus type 2. The following medications are listed on the client's medication record: metformin (Glucophage) 0.5 g po bid and repaglinide (Prandil) 1 mg po with meals. The morning blood glucose fingerstick is 98 mg/dl. Which action by the nurse is most appropriate?
   a. Hold the morning po medications.
   b. Give the metformin, but hold the repaglinide.
   c. Give the repaglinide, but hold the metformin.
   (d.) Give the po medications as ordered.

   Rationale: **(D) is the answer. The morning fingerstick result is WNL. Drug therapy should continue as ordered to maintain the blood glucose WNL. Options (a), (b), and (c) would not help the client remain in glycemic control.**

3. The client with end-stage renal disease is scheduled for hemodialysis in 2 hours. He has a L AV fistula and needs assistance with feeding. In delegating the care of the client, which nursing order is of priority?
   a. Feed the client first.
   b. Give all morning care before the dialysis.
   (c.) Take the blood pressure in the right arm.
   d. Feel for a vibration on the left arm.

   Rationale: **(C) is the answer. The AV fistula is the vascular access for the hemodialysis. Care must be taken not to occlude or cause trauma to the site. Options (a) and (b) are important but not the priority nursing order. Option (d) is part of the assessment process that is the responsibility of the professional nurse.**

Applying Critical Thinking Skills to Test Questions

INSTRUCTIONS: Circle the best answer for each test question. Write your rationale for selecting the answer. To enhance your learning and test taking skill, discuss your answer and rationale with a partner. The answer and the rationale can be found on the back of this page.

1. At 10:00 AM the nurse realizes that clonidine 0.1 mg po was administered to the wrong client at 9:00 AM. Which nursing action is of priority?
   a. Fill out an incident report.
   b. Notify the physician.
   c. Take the client's blood pressure.
   d. Take the vital signs of the client at noon.

   Rationale: ______________________________
   ____
   ____
   ____
   ____

2. A beta-blocking agent is added to the pharmacological therapy of a client with congestive heart failure. An expected therapeutic effect is
   a. a decrease in complaints of fatigue.
   b. a decrease in the heart rate.
   c. an increase in blood pressure.
   d. an increase in diuresis.

   Rationale: ______________________________
   ____
   ____
   ____
   ____

3. The client is taking hydrochorothiazide 25 mg po qd and is started on the ACE inhibitor, lisinopril 10 mg po qd. Which nursing intervention indicates the most appropriate follow through action?
   a. Monitor the client's output.
   b. Assess the client for impaired skin integrity.
   c. Assess the client's cardiac rhythm.
   d. Monitor the client's blood pressure.

   Rationale: ______________________________
   ____
   ____
   ____
   ____

Applying Critical Thinking Skills to Test Questions

HELPFUL HINTS: Read all test questions carefully. Identify key words in the question that will guide you in answering the question. In these test questions the **key words** to consider are **"priority," "expected therapeutic effect,"** and **"most appropriate."** Compare your rationale with the one in the test question.

1. At 10:00 AM the nurse realizes that clonidine 0.1 mg po was administered to the wrong client at 9:00 AM. Which nursing action is of priority?
   a. Fill out an incident report.
   b. Notify the physician.
   (c.) Take the client's blood pressure.
   d. Take the vital signs of the client at noon.

   Rationale: **(C) is the answer. Clonidine is a alpha-adrenergic agonist and blocking agent. After oral administration, clonidine begins to exert its effect within 1 hour. Option (a) is necessary, but assessing the client is priority. Option (b) is important, but it will be important to inform the physician of the current B/P. Option (d) is a good follow-up intervention, but not the priority intervention.**

2. A beta-blocking agent is added to the pharmacological therapy of a client with congestive heart failure. An expected therapeutic effect is
   a. a decrease in complaints of fatigue.
   (b.) a decrease in the heart rate.
   c. an increase in blood pressure.
   d. an increase in diuresis.

   Rationale: **(B) is the answer. Beta-blockers have multiple cardiac uses. The physiological effect is to decrease cardiac contractibility and workload. The client may experience an increase, rather than a decrease, in fatigue after beginning therapy–option (a). Options (c) and (d) do not address the mechanism of action of beta-blockers.**

3. The client is taking hydrochorothiazide 25 mg po qd and is started on the ACE inhibitor, lisinopril 10 mg po qd. Which nursing intervention indicates the most appropriate follow through action?
   a. Monitor the client's output.
   b. Assess the client for impaired skin integrity.
   c. Assess the client's cardiac rhythm.
   (d.) Monitor the client's blood pressure.

   Rationale: **(D) is the answer. The combination of drug therapy indicates the primary use is for the antihypertensive effects. Blood pressure should be monitored. Options (a), (b), and (c) do not address the effects of the combined drug therapy.**

Applying Critical Thinking Skills to Test Questions

INSTRUCTIONS: Circle the one best answer for each test question. Write your rationale for selecting the answer. To enhance your learning and test-taking skill, discuss your answer and rationale with a partner. The answer and the rationale can be found on the back of this page.

1. The home health nurse visits a client who has a history of congestive heart failure. The client is on enalapril, furosemide, and isosorbide. While talking with the client, the nurse notices that the client has a persistent dry, nonproductive cough. Which nursing action is most appropriate?
   a. Ask if the client is taking any cough medicine.
   b. Encourage the client to increase fluid intake.
   c. Ask if the client has experienced any chest pain.
   d. Notify the physician.

   Rationale: ____

2. The nurse is providing discharge instructions to an elderly client taking the following oral medications: wafarin 5 mg qd, furosemide 20 mg qd, and digoxin 25 mg qod. Which of the following is most important for the nurse to include in the instructions?
   a. "You can take the pills with meals."
   b. "Call the doctor if you notice any bruising."
   c. "Use a pill box to remind you of the medicines you need to take."
   d. "Take the furosemide in the morning that so you can sleep at night."

   Rationale: ____

3. The nurse is delegating the care of a stable client who had a chest tube inserted after complications with the insertion of a central subclavian line the night before. Which intervention is most important for the nurse to ask the nursing assistant to carry out?
   a. Count the respiratory rate for 1 full minute.
   b. Keep the client in a high-Fowler's position.
   c. Encourage the client to cough and deep breathe.
   d. Ask the client to remain in bed while the chest tube is in place.

   Rationale: ____

Applying Critical Thinking Skills to Test Questions

HELPFUL HINTS: Read all test questions carefully. Identify key words in the question that will guide you in answering the question. In these test questions the **key words** to consider are **"most appropriate"** and **"most important."** Compare your rationale with the one in the test question.

1. The home health nurse visits a client who has a history of congestive heart failure. The client is on enalapril, furosemide, and isosorbide. While talking with the client, the nurse notices that the client has a persistent dry, nonproductive cough. Which nursing action is most appropriate?
   a. Ask if the client is taking any cough medicine.
   b. Encourage the client to increase fluid intake.
   c. Ask if the client has experienced any chest pain.
   (d.) Notify the physician.

   Rationale: **(D) is the answer. A dry, nonproductive cough is a side effect of ACE inhibitors like enalapril. This may warrant a change in therapy. Options (a), (b), and (c) do not address this side effect.**

2. The nurse is providing discharge instructions to an elderly client taking the following oral medications: wafarin 5 mg qd, furosemide 20 mg qd, and digoxin 25 mg qod. Which of the following is most important for the nurse to include in the instructions?
   a. "You can take the pills with meals."
   (b) "Call the doctor if you notice any bruising."
   c. "Use a pill box to remind you of the medicines you need to take."
   d. "Take the furosemide in the morning that so you can sleep at night."

   Rationale: **(B) is the answer. Based on this situation, it is most important to teach the client to recognize signs of excessive anticoagulation therapy. Options (a) and (d) are good, but not the most important. Option (c) may not be the best since mixing digoxin with the other pills may be confusing for the elderly client if the digoxin needs to be held.**

3. The nurse is delegating the care of a stable client who had a chest tube inserted after complications with the insertion of a central subclavian line the night before. Which intervention is most important for the nurse to ask the nursing assistant to carry out?
   a. Count the respiratory rate for 1 full minute.
   b. Keep the client in a high-Fowler's position.
   (c.) Encourage the client to cough and deep breathe.
   d. Ask the client to remain in bed while the chest tube is in place.

   Rationale: **(C) is the answer. Clients with chest tubes should be encouraged to cough and deep breathe to enhance lung re-expansion. Options (a) and (b) are good but not the most important. Option (d) is not appropriate, and, unless contraindicated, the client should be encouraged to ambulate.**

Applying Critical Thinking Skills to Test Questions

INSTRUCTIONS: Circle the one best answer for each test question. Write your rationale for selecting the answer. To enhance your learning and test-taking skill, discuss your answer and rationale with a partner. The answer and the rationale can be found on the back of this page.

1. The client is on a heparin infusion after being diagnosed with a venous thrombus in the right leg. To best monitor the effect of the heparin therapy, the nurse would
   a. assess for signs and symptoms of bleeding.
   b. check the aPTT.
   c. monitor the PT.
   d. check the stool for occult blood.

   Rationale: ____

2. The nurse is assigned to a client who is 4 days post-op thoracic surgery and has a chest tube. The nurse learns in morning report that there has not been any drainage from the chest tube for the last 24 hours. In assessing the closed-chest drainage system, the nurse notes that there are no fluctuations in the water-seal chamber. The client's respirations are 22, unlabored. In planning the client care, the nurse would prepare
   a. for possible chest tube removal.
   b. for replacement of the chest tube.
   c. to increase the suction to the drainage system.
   d. to disconnect the chest tube from the drainage system.

   Rationale: ____

3. The nurse is caring for a client who is elderly, extremely confused, and restless this morning. The client is receiving oxygen, has a chest tube, and is continuously pulling at the tube. Which is the best plan of care for this client?
   a. Assign a staff RN to care for the client.
   b. Ask the nursing assistant to monitor the client and report changes.
   c. Assign a nursing assistant, but have the RN check the client q2h.
   d. Ask the LVN/LPN to care for the client and get an order for restraints.

   Rationale: ____

Applying Critical Thinking Skills to Test Questions

HELPFUL HINTS: : Read all test questions carefully. Identify key words in the question that will guide you in answering the question. In these test questions the **key words** to consider are **"best"** and **"planning the client care."** Compare your rationale with the one in the test question.

1. The client is on a heparin infusion after being diagnosed with a venous thrombus in the right leg. To best monitor the effect of the heparin therapy, the nurse would
   a. assess for signs and symptoms of bleeding.
   (b.) check the aPTT.
   c. monitor the PT.
   d. check the stool for occult blood.

   Rationale: **(B) is the answer. The aPTT (activated partial thromboplastin time) is used to monitor heparin therapy. Options (a) and (d) are good nursing interventions, but signs and symptoms are not the best indicators. Option (c) is mainly used to monitor wafarin therapy.**

2. The nurse is assigned to a client who is 4 days post-op thoracic surgery and has a chest tube. The nurse learns in morning report that there has not been any drainage from the chest tube for the last 24 hours. In assessing the closed-chest drainage system, the nurse notes that there are no fluctuations in the water-seal chamber. The client's respirations are 22, unlabored. In planning the client care, the nurse would prepare
   (a.) for possible chest tube removal.
   b. for replacement of the chest tube.
   c. to increase the suction to the drainage system.
   d. to disconnect the chest tube from the drainage system.

   Rationale: **(A) is the answer. The client is 4 days post-op. Respiratory signs indicate normal progression of lung re-expansion. Assessment findings do not support option (b). Options (c) and (d) demonstrate a need to review chest tubes and the drainage system.**

3. The nurse is caring for a client who is elderly, extremely confused, and restless this morning. The client is receiving oxygen, has a chest tube, and is continuously pulling at the tube. Which is the best plan of care for this client?
   (a.) Assign a staff RN to care for the client.
   b. Ask the nursing assistant to monitor the client and report changes.
   c. Assign a nursing assistant, but have the RN check the client q2h.
   d. Ask the LVN/LPN to care for the client and get an order for restraints.

   Rationale: **(A) is the answer. Clients whose medical condition is unstable should be assigned to the RN. The RN is the most appropriate person to assess and monitor for changes. Options (b) and (c) are not appropriate for this client who is medically unstable. Option (d) is not the best plan.**

Applying Critical Thinking Skills to Test Questions

INSTRUCTIONS: Circle the one best answer for each test question. Write your rationale for selecting the answer. To enhance your learning and test taking skill, discuss your answer and rationale with a partner. The answer and the rationale can be found on the back of this page.

1. The client is being treated with continuous heparin infusion for a pulmonary embolus. The morning result of the activated partial thromboplastin time is 100 sec (Control 30 sec). Which nursing intervention is of priority?
   a. Continue to monitor the client.
   b. Take the client's vital signs.
   c. Notify the physician.
   d. Check the previous result.

   Rationale: ____

2. The nurse is caring for a client who has a chest tube connected to a closed-chest drainage system with suction. In assessing the water-seal chamber, the nurse notes constant bubbling. Which nursing intervention is most appropriate?
   a. Document the findings.
   b. Continue to monitor the client.
   c. Check the chest tube for air leaks.
   d. Decrease the amount of suction.

   Rationale: ____

3. The nurse is totaling the chest tube output at 1400, the close of the shift. The chest tube drainage is at the 125 cc calibrated mark on the drainage device. The vertical tape along the side of the calibrated marks of the drainage device has a line drawn at 50 cc with the time of 0600. Which nursing intervention is most appropriate based on this finding?
   a. Draw a line at 125 cc and indicate 1400.
   b. Document 125 cc as the output for the shift.
   c. Assess the suction chamber for patency.
   d. Notify the charge nurse.

   Rationale: ____

Applying Critical Thinking Skills to Test Questions

HELPFUL HINTS: : Read all test questions carefully. Identify key words in the question that will guide you in answering the question. In these test questions the **key words** to consider are **"priority"** and **"most appropriate."** Compare your rationale with the one in the test question.

1. The client is being treated with continuous heparin infusion for a pulmonary embolus. The morning result of the activated partial thromboplastin time is 100 sec (Control 30 sec). Which nursing intervention is of priority?
   a. Continue to monitor the client.
   b. Take the client's vital signs.
   (c.) Notify the physician.
   d. Check the previous result.

   Rationale: **(C) is the answer. The goal of heparin infusion is to maintain the activated partial thromboplastin time (APTT) at 1.5 to 2 × the normal range. 100 sec is a critical value, and the client is at risk for bleeding. Options (a), (b), and (d) are good nursing interventions but not the priority intervention.**

2. The nurse is caring for a client who has a chest tube connected to a closed-chest drainage system with suction. In assessing the water-seal chamber, the nurse notes constant bubbling. Which nursing intervention is most appropriate?
   a. Document the findings.
   b. Continue to monitor the client.
   (c.) Check the chest tube for air leaks.
   d. Decrease the amount of suction.

   Rationale: **(C) is the answer. Constant bubbling in the water-seal chamber indicates an air leak. Options (a) and (b) are good interventions but are not the most appropriate based on the situation. Option (d) does not address the water-seal chamber.**

3. The nurse is totaling the chest tube output at 1400, the close of the shift. The chest tube drainage is at the 125-cc calibrated mark on the drainage device. The vertical tape along the side of the calibrated marks of the drainage device has a line drawn at 50 cc with the time of 0600. Which nursing intervention is most appropriate based on this finding?
   (a.) Draw a line at 125 cc and indicate 1400.
   b. Document 125 cc as the output for the shift.
   c. Assess the suction chamber for patency.
   d. Notify the charge nurse.

   Rationale: **(A) is the answer. The nurse monitors the chest tube drainage output by drawing a line at drainage level in the chamber at the end of the shift. Options (b), (c), and (d) are not appropriate interventions.**

Applying Critical Thinking Skills to Test Questions

INSTRUCTIONS: Circle the one best answer for each test question. Write your rationale for selecting the answer. To enhance your learning and test-taking skill, discuss your answer and rationale with a partner. The answer and the rationale can be found on the back of this page.

1. The nurse assesses the client who is 1 day post-op transurethral resection of the prostate. He has not had any output from the urinary catheter for 2 hours. The client has an order for intermittent bladder irrigation. Which technique is best for the nurse to use to safely carry out this order?
   a. Irrigate with 50 cc of sterile water and aspirate an equal amount of fluid.
   b. Use clean technique and irrigate until the return is free of clots.
   c. Use sterile technique and irrigate with 50 cc of solution at a time.
   d. Start a continuous bladder irrigation and infuse 200 cc over 30 minutes.

   Rationale: ____

   ____

   ____

   ____

   ____

2. The client has just experienced a generalized tonic-clonic type seizure in bed. Which nursing intervention is of priority immediately after the seizure?
   a. Document the findings.
   b. Maintain a quiet environment.
   c. Reorient the client to the surroundings.
   d. Position the client in a side-lying position.

   Rationale: ____

   ____

   ____

   ____

   ____

3. The nurse is assigned to a client who is 4 days post-op right hip replacement. The nurse finds the client eating breakfast, sitting comfortably in a chair with the right leg crossed over the left leg. Which nursing intervention is of priority?
   a. Assess the right hip dressing.
   b. Assess the client's pain level.
   c. Check the quality of the pedal pulses of both feet.
   d. Instruct the client to keep both feet flat on the floor.

   Rationale: ____

   ____

   ____

   ____

   ____

Applying Critical Thinking Skills to Test Questions

HELPFUL HINTS: Read all test questions carefully. Identify key words in the question that will guide you in answering the question. In these test questions the **key words** to consider are **"best"** and **"priority."** Compare your rationale with the one in the test question.

1. The nurse assesses the client who is 1 day post-op transurethral resection of the prostate. He has not had any output from the urinary catheter for 2 hours. The client has an order for intermittent bladder irrigation. Which technique is best for the nurse to use to safely carry out this order?
   a. Irrigate with 50 cc of sterile water and aspirate an equal amount of fluid.
   b. Use clean technique and irrigate until the return is free of clots.
   (c.) Use sterile technique and irrigate with 50 cc of solution at a time.
   d. Start a continuous bladder irrigation and infuse 200 cc over 30 minutes.

   Rationale: **(C) is the answer. Bladder irrigation is always performed using sterile technique. Solution is gently introduced into the bladder during irrigation. Options (a), (b), and (d) do not describe how to safely and correctly carry out this technique.**

2. The client has just experienced a generalized tonic-clonic type seizure in bed. Which nursing intervention is of priority immediately after the seizure?
   a. Document the findings.
   b. Maintain a quiet environment.
   c. Reorient the client to the surroundings.
   (d) Position the client in a side-lying position.

   Rationale: **(D) is the answer. Aspiration is a concern after the seizure since the client will be lethargic and oral secretions will need to be suctioned and allowed to drain. Options (a), (b), and (c) are good interventions but are not priority.**

3. The nurse is assigned to a client who is 4 days post-op right hip replacement. The nurse finds the client eating breakfast, sitting comfortably in a chair with the right leg crossed over the left leg. Which nursing intervention is of priority?
   a. Assess the right hip dressing.
   b. Assess the client's pain level.
   c. Check the quality of the pedal pulses of both feet.
   (d.) Instruct the client to keep both feet flat on the floor.

   Rationale: **(D) is the answer. Crossing of the feet or legs after hip replacement may put undue tension on the operative hip and increase the risk of hip dislocation. Options (a), (b), and (c) are good interventions but not priority.**

Applying Critical Thinking Skills to Test Questions

INSTRUCTIONS: Circle the one best answer for each test question. Write your rationale for selecting the answer. To enhance your learning and test-taking skill, discuss your answer and rationale with a partner. The answer and the rationale can be found on the back of this page.

1. The client is 4 days post-op colon resection and has an NG tube to low continuous suction. The client tells the nurse that he is feeling nauseated and then vomits 100 cc of yellow-green drainage. The nurse's initial action is to
   a. assess tube placement.
   b. administer an antiemetic.
   c. pull out the NG tube.
   d. increase the NG tube suction to moderate.

   Rationale: ______________________________

2. The client has been on full-strength formula tube feeding at 60 cc/hr via the NG tube for 2 days. In delegating the care of the client, which directive, given to the nursing assistant, most indicates that the nurse is monitoring for tube feeding complications?
   a. "Let me know if the client has liquid bowel movements this shift."
   b. "Weigh the client using the stand up scale as soon as report is over."
   c. "The client can sit in a chair for 30 minutes this morning."
   d. "Take the vital signs every 4 hours."

   Rationale: ______________________________

3. The physician orders to start continuous tube feedings at 50 ml/hr. After starting the tube feeding, it is most important for the nurse to initially plan to
   a. assess bowel sounds every shift.
   b. take the vital signs q4h.
   c. monitor residual q4h.
   d. monitor the intake and output.

   Rationale: ______________________________

Applying Critical Thinking Skills to Test Questions

HELPFUL HINTS: Read all test questions carefully. Identify key words in the question that will guide you in answering the question. In these test questions the **key words** to consider are **"initial,"** **"most indicates,"** and **"most important."** Compare your rationale with the one in the test question.

1. The client is 4 days post-op colon resection and has an NG tube to low continuous suction. The client tells the nurse that he is feeling nauseated and then vomits 100 cc of yellow-green drainage. The nurse's initial action is to
   (a.) assess tube placement.
   b. administer an antiemetic.
   c. pull out the NG tube.
   d. increase the NG tube suction to moderate.

   Rationale: **(A) is the answer. It is important to initially check the placement of the NG tube to ensure that the tube and suction are working. Option (b) may be performed if the N/V does not subside. Options (c) and (d) do not help to solve the problem.**

2. The client has been on full-strength formula tube feeding at 60 cc/hr via the NG tube for 2 days. In delegating the care of the client, which directive, given to the nursing assistant, most indicates that the nurse is monitoring for tube feeding complications?
   (a.) "Let me know if the client has liquid bowel movements this shift."
   b. "Weigh the client using the stand up scale as soon as report is over."
   c. "The client can sit in a chair for 30 minutes this morning."
   d. "Take the vital signs every 4 hours."

   Rationale: **(A) is the answer. Enteral feeding formulas can cause diarrhea. Option (b) helps to identify if the client is gaining weight. Options(c) and (d) are directives that promote good nursing care, but they are not directly related to identifying formula complications.**

3. The physician orders to start continuous tube feedings at 50 ml/hr. After starting the tube feeding, it is most important for the nurse to initially plan to
   a. assess bowel sounds every shift.
   b. take the vital signs q4h.
   (c.) monitor residual q4h.
   d. monitor the intake and output.

   Rationale: **(C) is the answer. Residual should be checked to ensure that the client is tolerating the tube feeding. Options (a), (b), and (d) are important but are not the most important.**

BIBLIOGRAPHY

Abrams, A. (2001). *Clinical Drug Therapy: Rationales for Nursing Practice.* (6th ed.). Philadelphia: Lippincott Williams & Wilkins.

Black, J., Hawks, J., & Keene, A. (2001). *Medical-Surgical Nursing: Clinical Management for Positive Outcomes.* (6th ed.). Philadelphia: W.B. Saunders Company.

Carpenito, L. (2002). *Nursing Diagnosis: Application to Clinical Practice.* (9th ed). Philadelphia: Lippincott Williams & Wilkins.

LeMone, P., & Burke, K. (2000). *Medical-Surgical Nursing: Critical Thinking in Client Care.* (2nd ed.). Englewood Cliffs, NJ: Prentice Hall, Inc.

Lilley, L., & Aucker, R. (2001). *Pharmacology and the Nursing Process.* (3rd ed.). St. Louis: Mosby.

Pagana, K., & Pagana, T. (2002). *Manual of Diagnostic and Laboratory Tests.* (2nd ed.). St. Louis: Mosby.

Phipps, W., Sands, J., & Marek, J. (1999). *Medical-Surgical Nursing: Concepts and Clinical Practice.* (6th ed.). St. Louis: Mosby.

Smeltzer, S., & Bare, B. (2000). *Medical-Surgical Nursing.* (9th ed.). Philadelphia: Lippincott Williams & Wilkins.

Taber's Cyclopedic Medical Dictionary. (2001) Philadelphia: F.A. Davis Company.